風呂

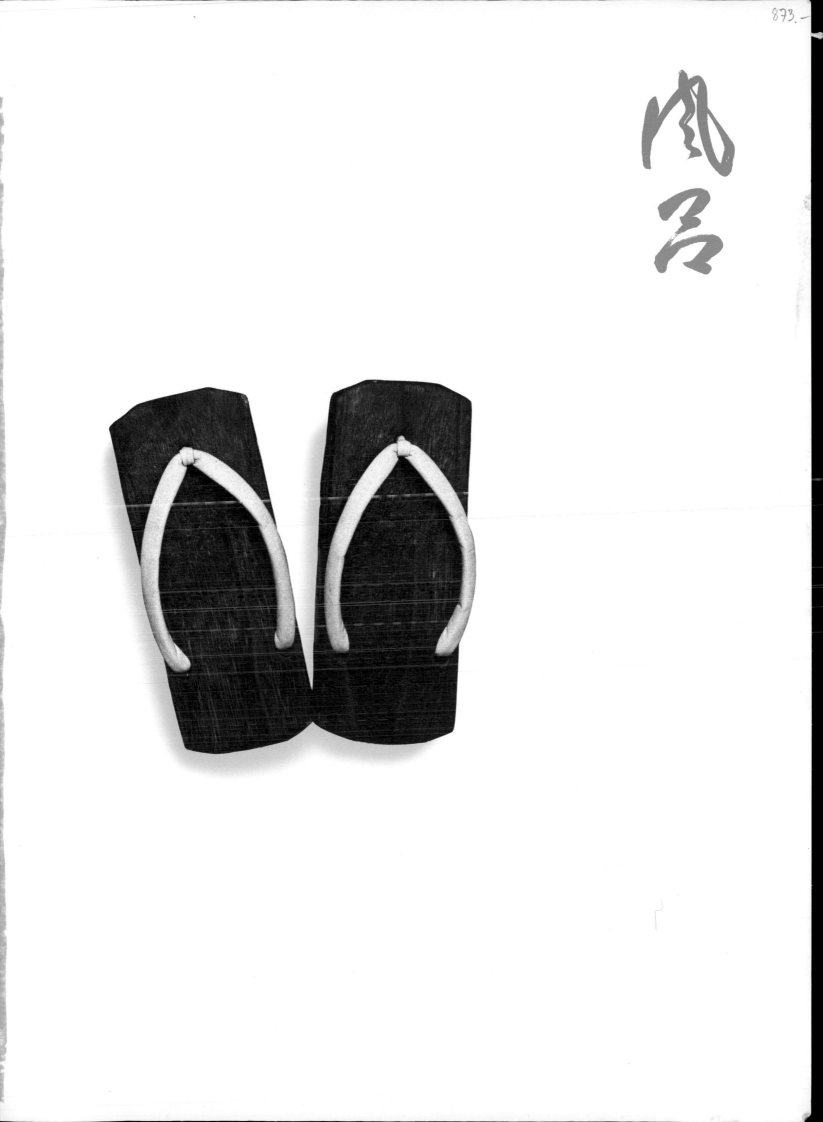

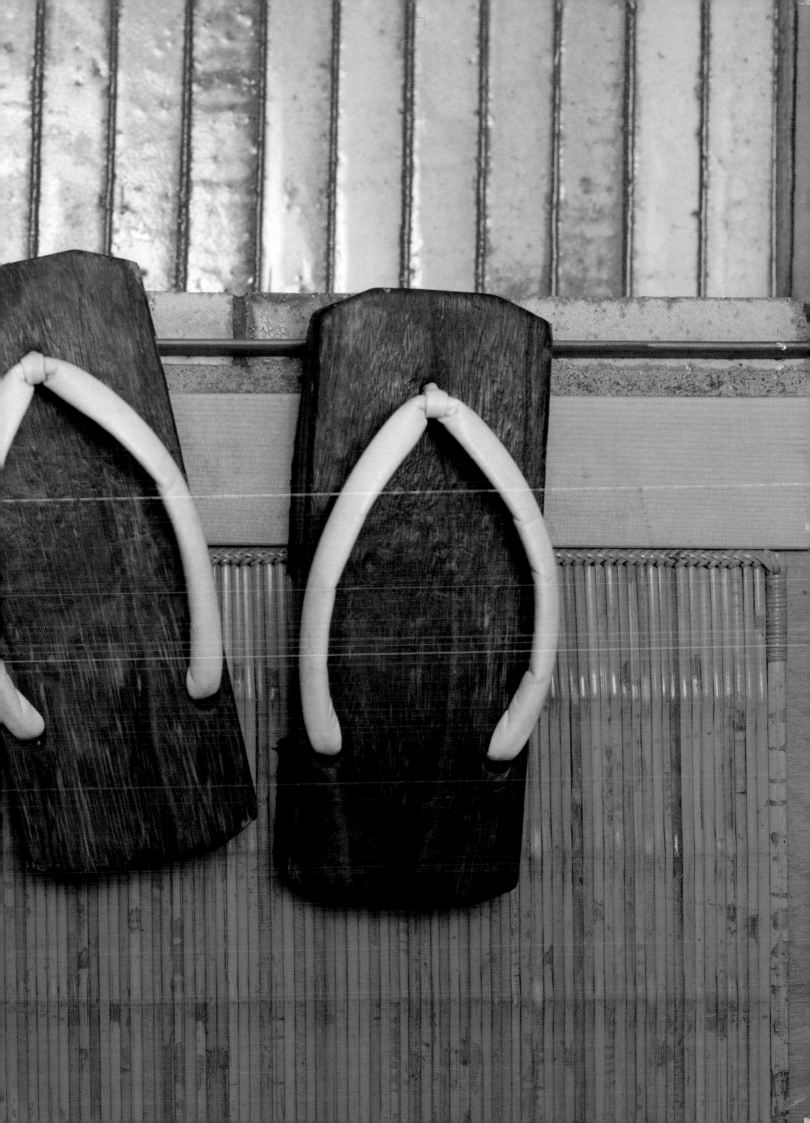

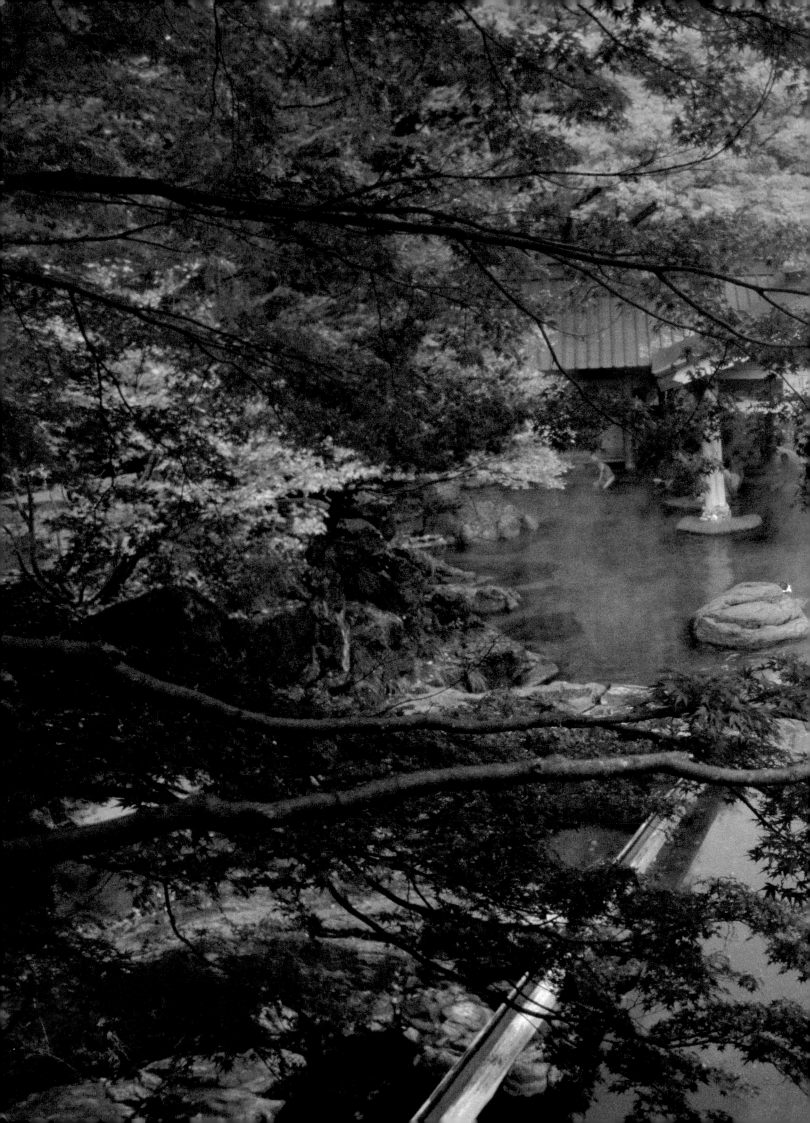

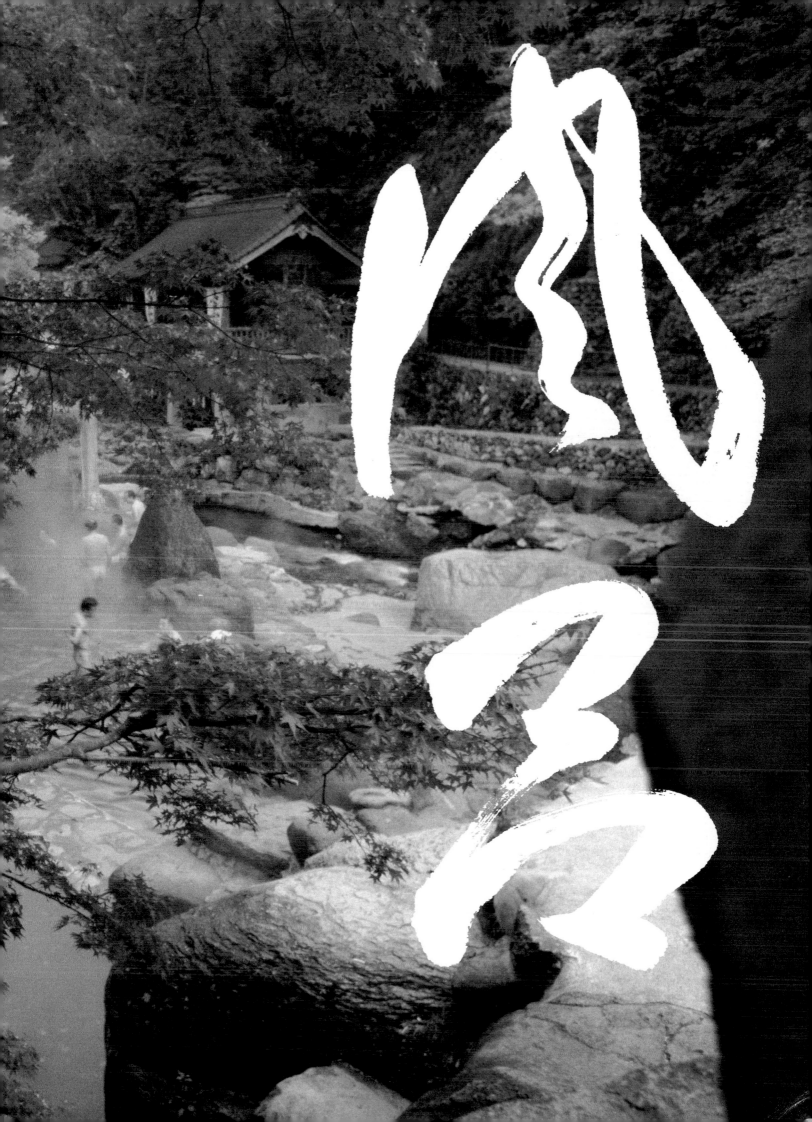

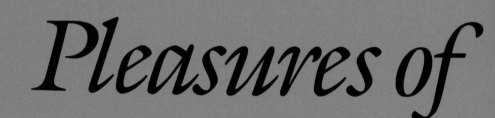

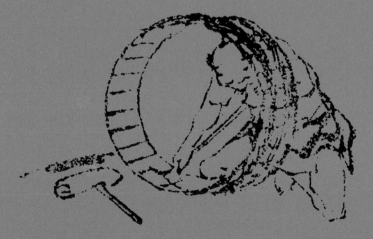

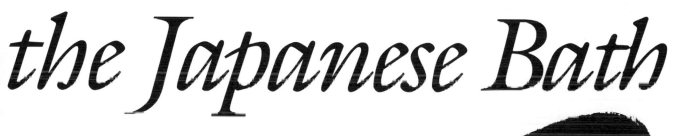

the Japanese Bath

text by
PETER GRILLI

photographs and design by
DANA LEVY

foreword by
ISAMU NOGUCHI

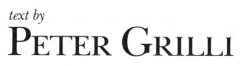

WEATHERHILLL
NEW YORK   TOKYO

COVER PHOTOGRAPHS

FRONT, TOP: Bathroom at Tawaraya Inn, Kyoto (p.166).

FRONT, BOTTOM: *Rotenburo* (open-air bath) at Shuzenji (p. 131).

BACK, TOP: Washing area at Urashima Hotel bathroom, Katsuura (p. 142).

BACK, BOTTOM: The "Cave of Forgotten Return," bath at Urashima Hotel,
Katsuura (p. 143).

CHAPTER OPENING PHOTOGRAPHS

Pp. 2-3: Wooden clogs *(geta)* left at entrance to a hot-spring bathhouse.

Pp. 4-5: The rustic hot-springs baths of the Chojukan Inn at Hoshi.

Pp. 6-7: The great open-air hot-spring pools at Takaragawa.

CHAPTER OPENING DECORATIONS

Sketches by Katsushika Hokusai, early nineteenth century (courtesy of
Ota Memorial Museum of Art).

Published by Weatherhill, Inc.
420 Madison Avenue, 15th Floor
New York 10017

First published in 1985 as *Furo: The Japanese Bath*
by Kodansha International Ltd.

Printed in Hong Kong

Library of Congress Cataloging in Publication Data

Grilli, Peter
    Pleasures of the Japanese bath / text by Peter Grilli;
photographs by Dana Levy; introduction by Isamu Noguchi.
       p.   cm.
    Includes index.
    ISBN 0-8348-0253-8: $24.95
    1. Bathing customs—Japan. 2. Baths—Japan. I. Title.
GT2846.J3G75 1992   92-4127
391'.64—dc20   CIP

Citations in this book (on the pages indicated) are from the following sources: pp. 46–
47, *The Kojiki: Records of Ancient Matters*, translated by Basil Hall Chamberlain (Tokyo:
Charles E. Tuttle, 1981); pp. 26, 48, *Meeting With Japan*, by Fosco Maraini (New York:
Viking Press, 1960); pp. 55–56, *The Three Treasures: A Study and Translation of Minamoto
Tamenori's Sanboe*, by Edward Burt Kamens (Ann Arbor, Mich.: Center for Japanese
Studies, University of Michigan, forthcoming), by permission; p. 59, *The Pillow Book of
Sei Shonagon*, translated by Ivan Morris (New York: Columbia University Press, 1967), by
permission; pp. 61–62, *Murasaki Shikibu: Her Diary and Poetic Memoirs*, translated by
Richard Bowring (Princeton, N.J.: Princeton University Press, 1982), by permission; pp.
64–66, *The Tale of the Heike*, translated by Hiroshi Kitagawa and Bruce T. Tsuchida (To-
kyo: University of Tokyo Press, 1975), by permission; pp. 66–67, *The Hagakure*, by
Yamamoto Tametomo, translated by Takao Mukoh (Tokyo: Hokuseido Press, 1980), by
permission; pp. 68–69, *They Came to Japan: An Anthology of European Reports on Japan,
1543–1640*, compiled by Michael Cooper (Berkeley, Calif.: University of California
Press, 1965); pp. 80–83, *Shikitei Sanba and the Comic Tradition in Edo Fiction*, by Robert
Leutner (Cambridge, Mass.: Harvard-Yenching Institute, 1985), by permission; p. 141
(chart), *Sensual Water*, by Bernard Barber and Dana Levy (Chicago: Contemporary
Books, 1978), by permission; pp. 144–48, *The Three-Cornered World* (Japanese title:
Kusamakura), by Natsume Soseki, translated by Alan Turney (London: Peter Owen,
1965), by permission; pp. 166–68, *Japanese Homes and Their Surroundings*, by Edward
Sylvester Morse (New York: Dover, 1961).

NOTE: The names of Japanese figures active before 1868 are given in Japanese order,
with surname first; those of subsequent eras are given in Western order.

Contents

For Susan and Tish
Our Companions of the Bath

by Isamu Noguchi

13

Ultimately, to be in Japan is to enter the *furo* again—to shed one's workday clothes, bathe leisurely, and don a comfortable, household *yukata* before dinner. The great potter Rosanjin, for one, would insist on doing this before his afternoon beer so he could watch the best time of day settle into dusk from the vantage point of his tub. Six o'clock was not an unusual hour for dining, especially in the countryside. But times have changed.

The classic *furo* was a box of *hinoki* wood, sacred and fragrant, with a fire chamber set into one end. The fire was fed from the outside with twigs to transform the water into *o-yu* (hot water)—a gradual, time-consuming process. So the bath fire was lit early, allowing time for a leisurely soak that would keep one warm till bedtime. The same was true of the public bath and the *onsen* (hot-spring bath), where the heat is of so penetrating a sort as to act as a blanket, like it or not. At such places, too, one bathed in the afternoon. For that matter, even when invited to a friend's house, perhaps to see his collection, one would go no later than three o'clock, first to enter his *furo* and cleanse oneself of the outside world in preparation for the long afternoon's flow into evening, with all the stages of food tasting and art viewing in between.

As for the quality of the *o-yu* itself, I am of the opinion that the *goemon-buro* is the best. This round tub is a cauldron of cast iron, about a yard in diameter and height, heated by a fire built directly beneath it. Inside the tub, the body is precariously balanced on a floating wooden lid that gradually sinks to the bottom under one's weight, while the heat and bubbles rise from below. No one bathes in a *goemon-buro* nowadays except for a few connoisseurs in the countryside. There is room in this type of *furo* for only one person at a time, and an assistant is needed to maneuver the water scoop and replenish water gently poured over one's back. What would Japan do without people at every turn?

And what can one do to avoid unwanted surprises such as that I experienced the other day when caught overnight at a business hotel at Narita Airport. I found myself squeezed into a pink plastic box that masqueraded as a *furo*. Throughout the room not even an illusion of time or space remained, only a crowd of things from bed to television as if to make any other description of Japan today a lie. Perhaps this is the logical, if ironic, result of the new architecture, with people reconciled to no time, no space, self-sufficient with their modern conveniences while they busily concern themselves with trying to recall the past, with learning about the poetry of Basho and the more elegant customs of the Heian court.

It is the *furo* and the *o-yu* that help us remember. Even in our cramped little modern tubs, submerged to our necks in hot water, we luxuriate in our memories of time and space, and feel ourselves alive once again.

Few visitors to Japan fail to remark on the extraordinary Japanese passion for bathing. The early Chinese historians commenting in the third century A.D. on the peculiar habits of their primitive island neighbors to the east, the Christian missionaries and traders of the sixteenth and seventeenth centuries, and foreign tourists, soldiers, students, and businessmen of the present day—all have quickly taken note of the Japanese penchant for frequent bathing, their custom of bathing communally, and their delight in soaking in waters so hot as to seem beyond human tolerance. Bolstered by the obvious pleasure of Japanese bathers, courage generally follows quickly upon initial curiosity. Foreigners are soon persuaded to take the plunge themselves; by the time they rise refreshed from the delicious lassitude of their first soak in a Japanese tub, most visitors are converts.

To some, the Japanese bath approaches a religious experience. To others, its chief purpose is sensual gratification. Some turn to the bath seeking a cure for the most severe disorders of the body. Still others find in it a means of treating the afflictions of the spirit far more effective than the analytical approaches of Western Freudians. Like the elephant that represented all things to the five blind men examining it, the Japanese bath offers a multitude of blessings to those who partake of its special pleasures.

For students of comparative culture, the bath offers a useful point of reference in contrasting Japanese and Western attitudes. In the West today, we tend to regard bathing as a private, domestic affair—a means of keeping clean and free of disease—and little more. Although our culture retains vestiges of ancient beliefs regarding ritual purification—baptismal ceremonies, sprinkling of holy water, and the like—bathing in the West is not invested with the religious significance it has had in Japan since ancient times. To us, bathing is a solitary business, taking place at home, for the most part, and behind closed doors. To the Japanese, bathing at its best is a communal activity, where individuals reinforce familial or social ties by sharing a tub or by scrubbing each other's backs. Public bathhouses in Japanese cities have played a role as community gathering places for the last four hundred years, comparable to the central plazas or coffee houses of European towns—centers where neighbors could meet regularly to share news and gossip. Our bathrooms tend to be small, rather confining spaces, clean in an antiseptic way and lacking any of the aesthetic flourishes or comforts that we lavish on other rooms in the house that we distinguish as "living" quarters. Baths in Japanese homes are much better integrated into the living spaces of the household. Though small, they are often beautifully appointed—in wealthier homes, with wooden paneling and a tub finely handcrafted from aromatic cypress wood—and may face a courtyard garden designed to be viewed while soaking in the tub.

Western attitudes toward bathing have not always been so far removed from those of Japan. The pre-Christian Mediterranean cultures of Egypt, Greece, and Rome shared similar notions of the congruence of spiritual health with physical cleanliness. In those societies, too, bathing was often a luxurious communal affair, as testified by the ruins of huge bathing emporia in Rome, Pompeii, and Bath, as well as in North Africa, Asia Minor, and other parts of the Roman Empire. Inhibitions about public nudity seem not to have concerned inhabitants of the ancient Mediterranean world, as they have not the Japanese until relatively recent times.

Today in America, we are beginning to relearn the lessons of the Romans and to appreciate the wisdom never forgotten by the Japanese. Surely, our increasing passion for hot tubs and whirlpool baths and our rapidly relaxing inhibitions about our bodies owe as much to the example of Japan as to the sexual revolution. It is to be hoped that these will not prove to be mere passing fads but will become lasting elements in a larger, ongoing effort to deepen and enrich the meaning of life.

This book developed out of the many hours of pleasant reflection spent in baths all over Japan. My earliest memory of Japan, as a child of five years, is the hot-spring pools at the resort of Unzen near Nagasaki. No doubt the experience of splashing about in those sulphurous waters at that tender age instilled in me, as it must in most Japanese children, a love of the hot-spring experience that only became keener as I grew older and visited more and more spas throughout the country. By now it has become an addiction. Japanese travel guidebooks identify more than two thousand hot springs large enough to have at least one hostelry, and thousands more that are simple, undeveloped natural springs far from overnight accommodations except a nearby farmhouse, perhaps, or a spot to pitch a tent. I have visited some two hundred hot springs in my years in Japan. If I am lucky, maybe I'll get to all of them.

Though this book may have been inspired by a long, pleasurable soak in some warm mountain pool, it is not solely about Japan's hot springs. Equal attention has been given to domestic baths, to the various types of communal baths, and to the story of the development of Japanese bathing habits. I have tried to write about the Japanese bath as a microcosm of many features of Japanese life and history. This may seem odd to someone who thinks of bathing as little more than a necessary social habit, a bit of a time-consuming nuisance, perhaps, but an unavoidable requirement for health and cleanliness. The Japanese do not think about bathing that way at all, and their attitudes toward bathing can be revealing about their attitudes toward life, society, and many other things. A religious history of Japan as seen through the bath is not inconceivable. Similarly, a social history of Japan as seen through the bath might also be written. So could a treatise on Japanese psychology, or a study of Japanese popular entertainment. I was not ambitious enough to undertake any of these studies, but reflections on all these themes run through this collection of words and images on the bath in Japan.

In researching the role of the bath in Japanese history and in present-day society, I learned much from the writings of many Japanese individuals whose published work inspired and guided my own study. Chief among these are Kunio Yanagida, Eizo Nakano, Ryuichi Tamura, Kazue Morisaki , Katsuzo Takeda, Mineo Hashimoto, Norio Ozaki, and Goichi Fujinami. Japanese travel-oriented periodicals and guidebooks offer a wealth of information about hot springs, and I am indebted to the many anonymous researchers and editors who compile the extensive literature issued by such publishers as Japan Travel Bureau, Ryoko Yomiuri Shuppansha, Akatsuki Kyoiku Tosho, Fujin Seikatsu-sha, and Jitsugyo no Nihon Sha.

Without the contributions of many other individuals, Japanese and otherwise, this book would have been impossible—or at least far more difficult—to complete. Some introduced Dana Levy and myself to unfamiliar hot springs that we might otherwise have not investigated; others opened their private baths or their inns to our cameras and inquiries; friends intrigued by the subject directed us to sources of information or illustrations that had eluded us; and still others aided in ways too informal or too personal to be described in detail here. Although the long list that follows must be impersonally alphabetical, each person named in it knows the special way in which he or she contributed to this book, and each should be aware as well of the warm gratitude of its authors: Tadashi Akaishi, Virginia Atchley, Bernard Barber, Raymond Bushell, Ann Harakawa, Fred Harris, Rev. Mineo Hashimoto, Sachiko Kagoshima, Tetsuo Kinoshita, Zenzo Matsuyama, Okinori Murata, Kenn Nakamura, Yoshiaki Nakamura, Kentaro Nakaya, Saburo Nobuki, Isamu Noguchi, Letitia O'Connor, Ryuzo Okamura, Seiichi Otsuka, Pamela Pasti, Matsuno Patrick, Jean Pearce, Donald Richie, Katsuhiko Sakiyama, Patricia Salmon, Emily Sano, Toshi Sato, Oliver Statler, Patricia Storandt, Hideko Takamine, Toru and Asaka Takemitsu, craftsmen of the Tarugen shop, staff of the Tawaraya Inn, Meredith Weatherby, Hidetoshi Yamaguchi, and Junsei Yamaguchi.

       For so visual a subject as baths and bathing in Japan, a book like this would be inconceivable without illustrations and text working together in a seamless harmony. I am deeply indebted to Dana Levy for creating this book. Not only did he produce the many, many superb photographs (as if that were not achievement enough, given the steamy conditions of bathing places and the often suspicious glares of other bathers), but he also conceived the very idea of the book and constantly urged me on in trying to find words to accompany his images even when they needed none at all. It was Dana also who found most of the illustrations by Japanese painters and woodcut artists. Finally, it was his talent as a book designer that combined the prints and paintings with his own photographs into a beautifully illumined whole. Our close relationship has made for an excellent collaboration in every sense of the word: mutually reinforcing, mutually critical, and mutually satisfying.

       Finally, to my wife, Susan, I am endlessly grateful for her inspiration and encouragement. Her response to baths and hot springs on her very first visit to Japan was so immediately positive that it convinced me of the value of a book such as this. It was often through her enthusiastic reactions to places I had visited long ago that I rediscovered their beauty or excitement. It was through the intuitive friendships that she, a foreigner speaking virtually no Japanese, struck up in the baths that I came to realize fully what the Japanese mean by "skinship." And it was through her determination to reproduce at home in the United States the Japanese bath experience that I finally recognized the benefits that it offers to anyone, anywhere.

Pleasures of the Japanese Bath

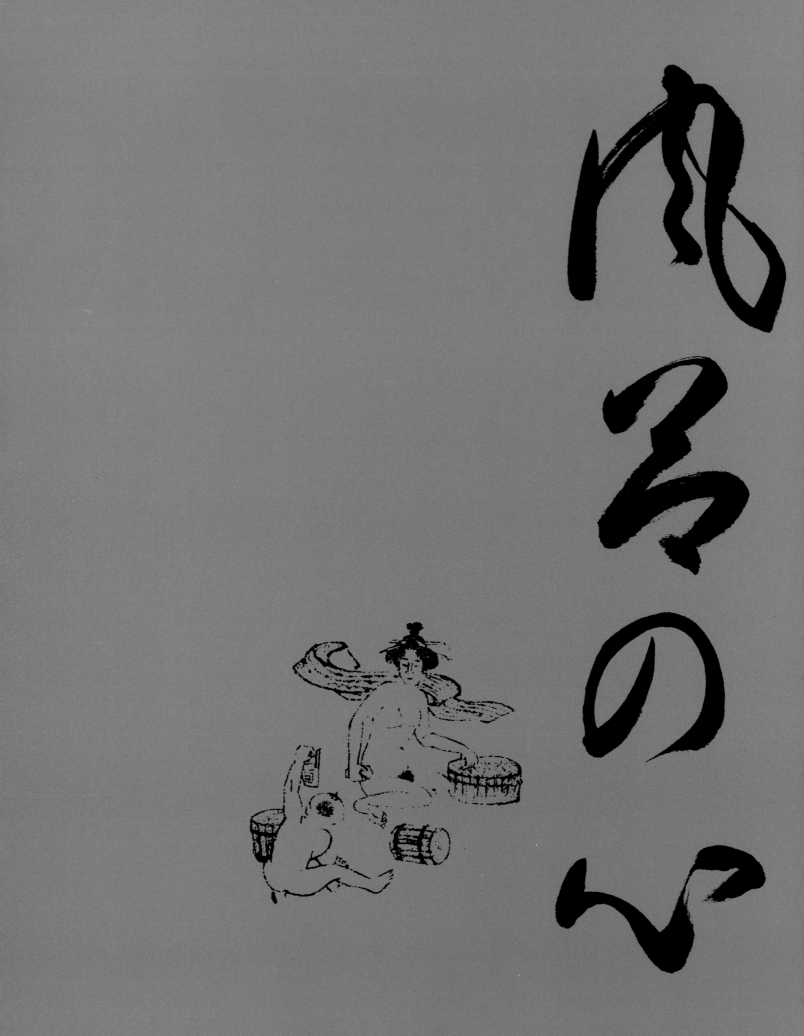

CHAPTER ONE

The Spirit of the Bath

*F*ew peoples have delighted in bathing as much as the Japanese, blessed since the earliest times with abundant hot water from mineral springs located throughout their volcanic land. Indeed, it is impossible to imagine a time when the Japanese were unaware of the sensual pleasures of the bath, to say nothing of its practical hygienic benefits. In places where hot-spring water was not readily available, whatever fuel was at hand was dedicated first to heating hot water for bathing, which took precedence over the needs of cooking food or heating homes: food could be eaten raw—indeed it was usually considered better that way—and in Japan's relatively temperate climate, the heating of dwellings was rarely a requirement for survival. But bathing was, and is.

At its simplest, the Japanese bath is merely a way of getting clean. But even a single experience reveals that it is also much more than that. After rinsing away the grime of everyday life outside the tub, one slips slowly into a deep pool or tub of sparkling clean hot water and sits submerged to the chin. Only a few minutes of soaking in that water, its heat seeping deep into the body, and the mind begins to drift. Is it the heat?

The public baths of Edo provided continuous inspiration for the facile and inventive brush of Katsushika Hokusai. The *Hokusai Manga*, a series of sketchbooks, abounds in drawings of nude figures bathing, many of which were later translated into more complex compositions in the prints of this extraordinarily productive artist. (*Courtesy of Ota Museum of Art*)

22   The depth? The steam? Or the sensation of floating while sitting immobile? Whatever the cause, all anguish, tension, anger, or pain seems to evaporate, replaced by a sublime euphoria. This is what the Japanese have known for millennia: that the bath offers a good deal more than functional hygiene.

The process of getting clean is, in itself, less what concerns the Japanese than the spirit of cleanliness. If the only purpose of bathing were simply to become clean, a shower would certainly work as well. But few Japanese today, even those who are thoroughly modern in other respects, would willingly exchange their tub for a shower, despite the undeniable advantages offered by the newfangled device; speed and efficiency are not at all what bathing is about in the Japanese mind. Similarly, if the Japanese bathed only to rid themselves of dirt, it would not be necessary to adhere quite so faithfully to a regimen of daily baths. But the motivations for bathing in Japan go beyond efficiency and transcend physical cleanliness. What the bath offers is a sensual feeling of well-being, of harmony with one's environment and with one's self. The delicious lassitude that overcomes the bather's spirit as he sits long and happily in a hot tub fosters a sense of generous tolerance. Along with relieving the pain of physical wounds or aching muscles, the bath also dispels the disorders of an uneasy mind, replacing them with a sense of calm and harmonious integration. Anger and frustration disappear and one's spirit returns to what must have been the peaceful innocence of the womb. For, as numerous sayings have proclaimed, in the bath not only does the Japanese wash his body, he cleanses his soul.

The Japanese are, of course, not unique in cherishing the pleasures of the bath. In the West, in the pre-Christian days of Egypt, Greece, and Rome, bathing was equally valued for the spiritual refreshment it imparted along with the utilitarian benefit of warding off disease. After the fall of Rome, the Turks perpetuated the steam baths of the Greeks and Romans and spread them throughout the Middle East. The Russians and Scandinavians have similarly found health and spiritual well-being in their saunas. But surely the Japanese are

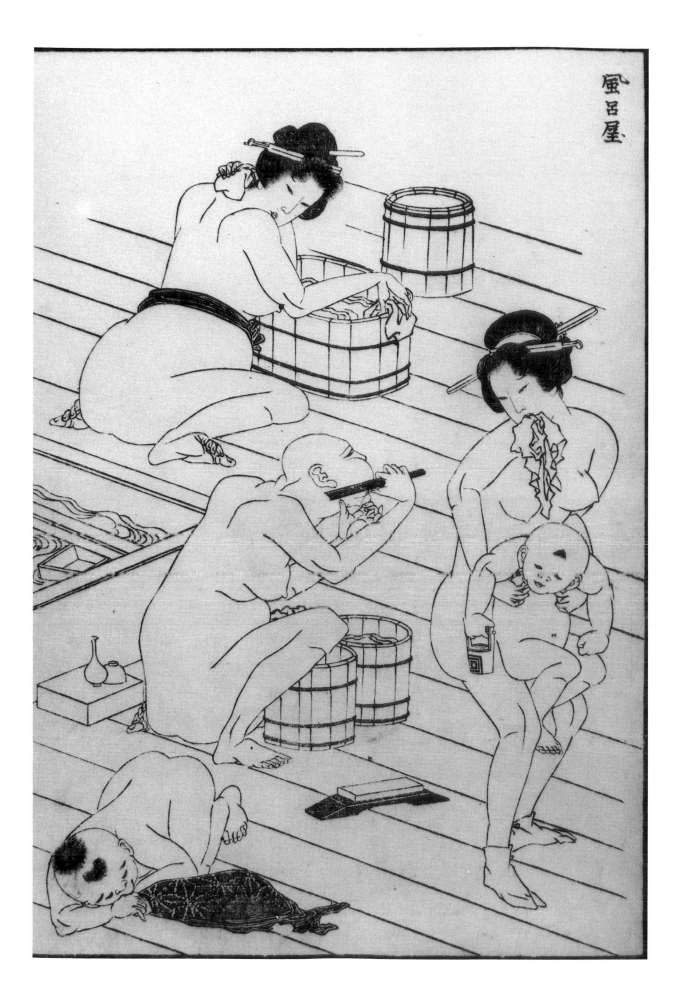

風呂屋

Bathers at the indoor "jungle baths" at Ibusuki revel in the illusion that they are in rocky mountain cascades or other such wild outdoor settings.

unequaled in their preoccupation with bathing and in the artistry they have lavished on the accoutrements of the bath.

"Cleanliness is next to godliness," John Wesley is said to have reminded his eighteenth-century parishioners, quoting ancient Hebrew scripture. But until relatively recently in the Christian era, Western societies have paid that dictum more lip service than actual observance. The Japanese need no such exhortations: they have known, believed, and practiced this truism from the earliest moments of their cultural identity. It is no exaggeration to say that they have made a religion of cleanliness, for the implications of ritual purification pervade the most ancient Shinto ethos and have remained constant throughout the development of Japanese cultural history. The earliest myths of the Japanese people refer repeatedly to acts of bathing or ritual lustration by the gods as they carried out their tasks of creating the universe and setting the heavenly and earthly societies in order. Indeed, the central deities of the ancient Shinto cosmos—the gods of sun, moon, and agricultural fertility— were all born out of a bath in which Izanagi, the ultimate creator-ancestor, washed his body.

In the Shinto tradition, evil and immorality have always been associated with filth and impurity, and virtue with cleanliness. This ethical principle has retained its literal as well as figurative vitality throughout Japanese cultural history and has colored all aspects of Japanese life. Described as the "Shinto attitude" for lack of a better term, the notions of natural purity, simplicity, and aesthetic as well as physical cleanliness have influenced all Japanese designs for living: art and architecture, literature and self-expression, the preparation of food, patterns of familial and societal organization, craft and productivity—in short, all activities by which man defines his existence and orders his life. To attribute to Japanese habits of bathing a causal role in the development of other such cultural patterns may be to give them far too weighty a responsibility, but it is perfectly appropriate to integrate these habits into the overall ethos that goes by the name Shinto. If Shinto is seen as a kind of continuous cultural thread linking present-day sensibilities to

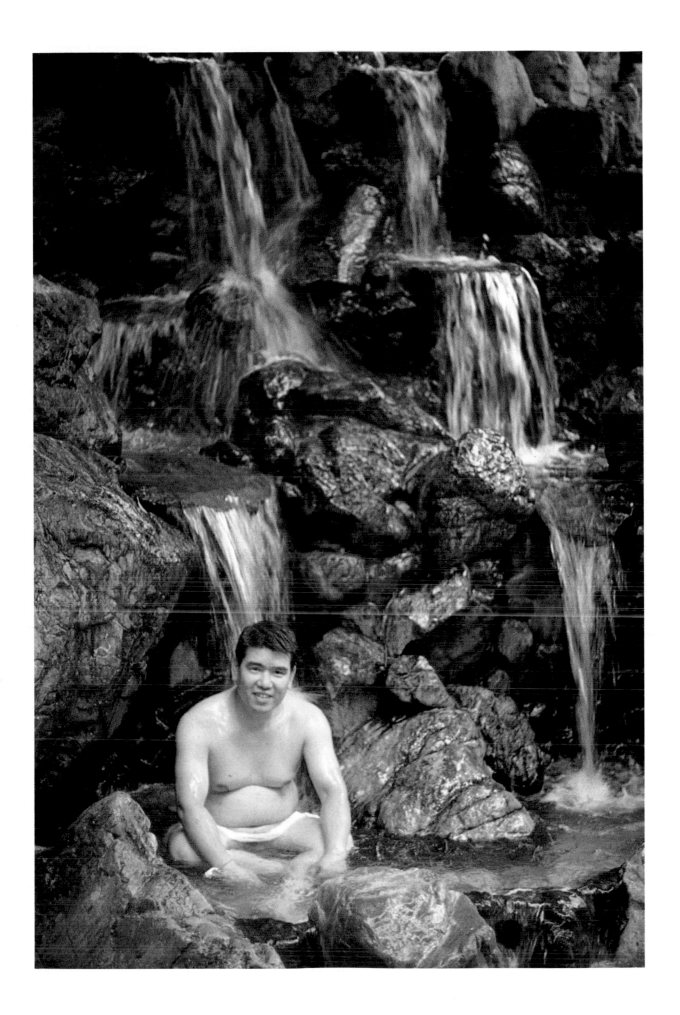

The relaxation afforded by a soak
in the natural hot water of a
geothermal spring induces revelry
and high spirits. Here, a group of
young office workers enjoys an
outing at a rural hot spring.

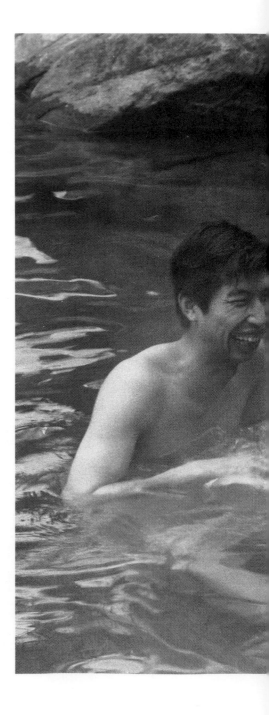

26   ancient animism and ancestor worship, then the bath may be
regarded as an important manifestation of the desire for purity
that characterizes all aspects of the Shinto view of the world. As
Fosco Maraini has put it, "In Japan, the ultimate origins of the
bath are religious. The bath is a domestic aspect of ancient puri-
ficatory rites *(yuami, misogi)* which from the earliest times were
an essential element of the Shinto cult."

It is remarkable how little bathing practices
have changed over the two thousand years or so of Japanese history, especially considering that the culture experienced periods
of abrupt and drastic transformation due to intense influence
from abroad. At two such moments in Japan's cultural history—
the importation of Buddhism and Chinese culture in the sixth
and seventh centuries, and the period of intense Westernization
that followed the Meiji Restoration of 1868—virtually every
aspect of traditional life was reexamined, tested against alternative foreign modes of behavior, and in many instances dis-
carded. From dressing habits to religious beliefs to patterns of
political organization, nearly everything foreign was seen as
superior to its Japanese counterpart, with the result that Japanese culture was transformed and redesigned according to new
models. But despite the faddish and often headlong rush to
adopt new patterns of dress, thought, and behavior, the Japanese have always been too pragmatic to abandon those things of
their own that they found most comfortable and that seemed to
work best. Thus did their bath remain virtually unchanged
through the ages. When something is perfect, after all, only a
fool would try to improve on it.

Inevitably, however, some changes and improve-
ments in peripheral aspects of the bath have taken place: as the
technology developed to provide city dwellers with the large
quantities of hot water previously available only at natural hot
springs, steam baths (which required less hot water) gradually
gave way in urban bathhouses to large, deep tanks of hot water;
modern plumbing systems rendered obsolete the old practices
of hauling water bucketful by bucketful or sending it through
primitive bamboo pipes. Today, mass-produced containers of

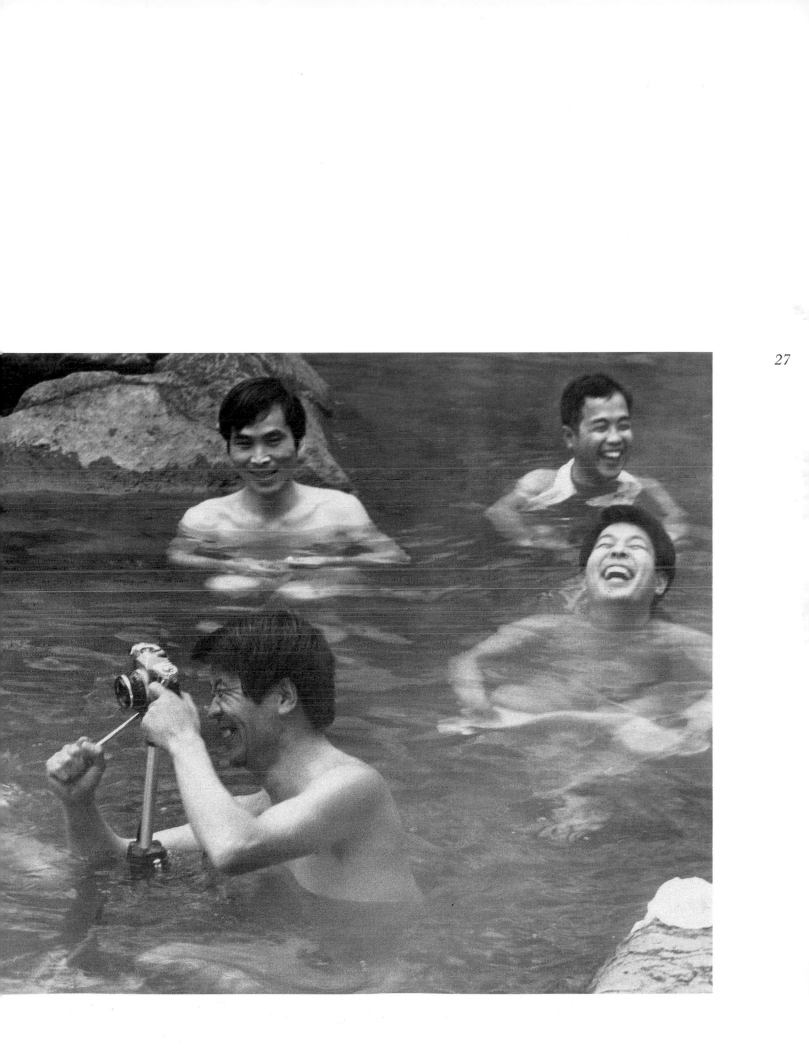

Baths and bathers throughout the centuries. *Below, clockwise from upper left:* Torii Kiyonaga, *The Bathroom,* c. 1780 (*Courtesy of Keio University*); artist unknown, *Bathers in a Steam Bath*; Yuki Ogura, *Two Bathers,* 1938 (*Courtesy of National Museum of Modern Art, Tokyo*); Utagawa Yoshiiku, *Battle in the Bathhouse,* c. 1868 (*Courtesy of Maspro Denkoh Art Gallery*). *Opposite:* A contemplative bather at the Tawaraya Inn, Kyoto.

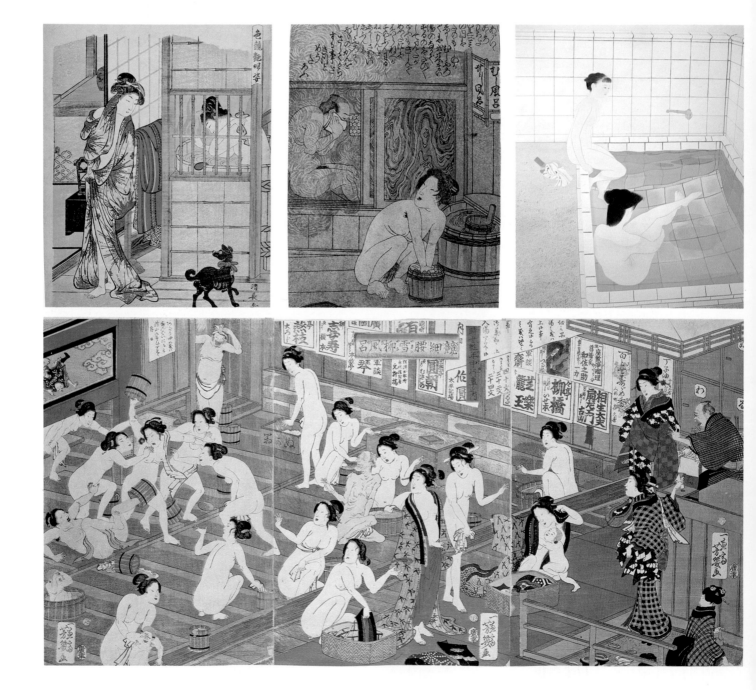

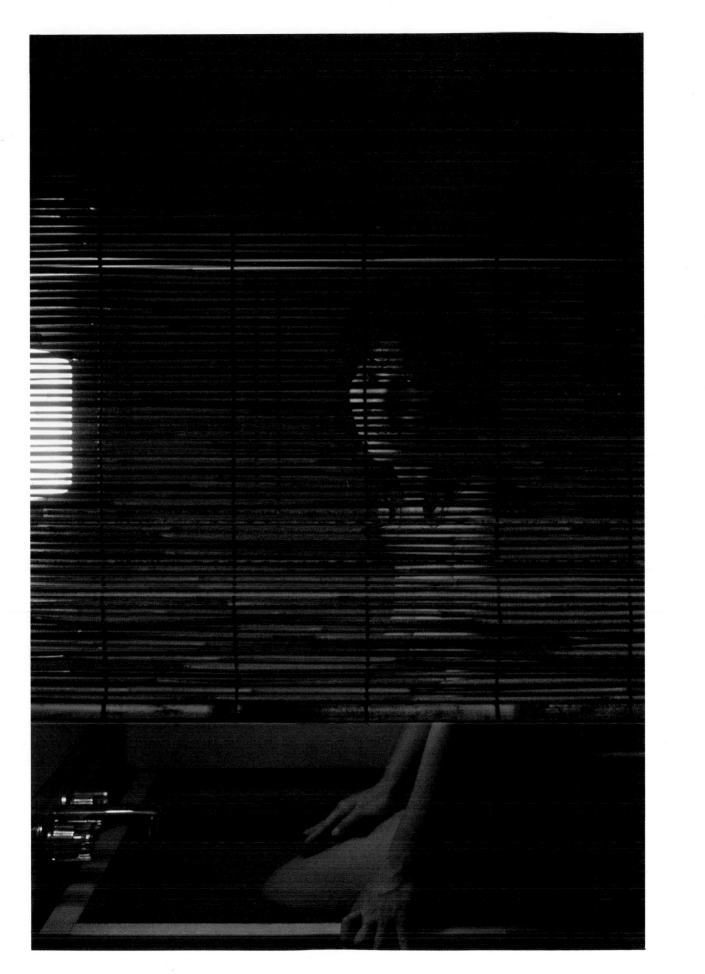

Life imitates art in the "jungle
bath" at Ibusuki.

metal, tile, or plastic have largely replaced the beautifully
handcrafted tubs of wood. Nevertheless, the habit of bathing
daily and the practice of washing away body dirt outside the tub
and enjoying a long relaxing soak in a deep tub or pool of clean
hot water have continued unaltered through the centuries.

The sensual pleasures of soaking in a Japanese
bathtub indoors are further enhanced by repeating the experience outdoors. Any visitor to a hot-spring resort will quickly
attest to the special delights of soaking in a *rotenburo*—a large
natural hot-spring pool exposed to the open sky. For it is there
that the bather slips peacefully into a sense of gentle harmony
with his natural surroundings. Succumbing to the drowsiness
brought on by leisurely immersion in the hot water, he drifts in a
half-sleep, oblivious to the fretful concerns of everyday affairs
and yet attuned to the trickle of the brook nearby, the rustling of
leaves, and the chirping of birds overhead. In winter, when the
sounds of nature are muted by a blanket of snow, the appeal of a
rotenburo bath is even greater. Soaking in the soothing hot water
that bubbles up from the earth, the bather is immune to the
crisp frostiness of the air; and when he rises steaming from the
outdoor pool, he carries its warmth with him, deep inside his
body.

As proof of these effects one need only watch a
party of Japanese bathers at a large open-air hot spring. First,
they splash about boisterously, loudly exclaiming about their
pleasure and slyly sneaking peeks at other bathers. But before
long, they grow quieter and one after another slump deeper
into the hot water. They speak less and less, but breathe deeply
and emit occasional moans of grateful pleasure. Slowly a cloud
of subconscious enlightenment seems to envelop their spirits,
beckoning them closer toward a feeling of unity with the rocks
and water, the trees and sky around them.

Bathing in Japan is best when it is communal.
Never inhibited by the Judeo-Christian embarrassment about
the human body or taboos on public nudity, the Japanese have
always bathed in groups. Until quite recently, men and women
soaked together in public bathhouses as well as hot springs.

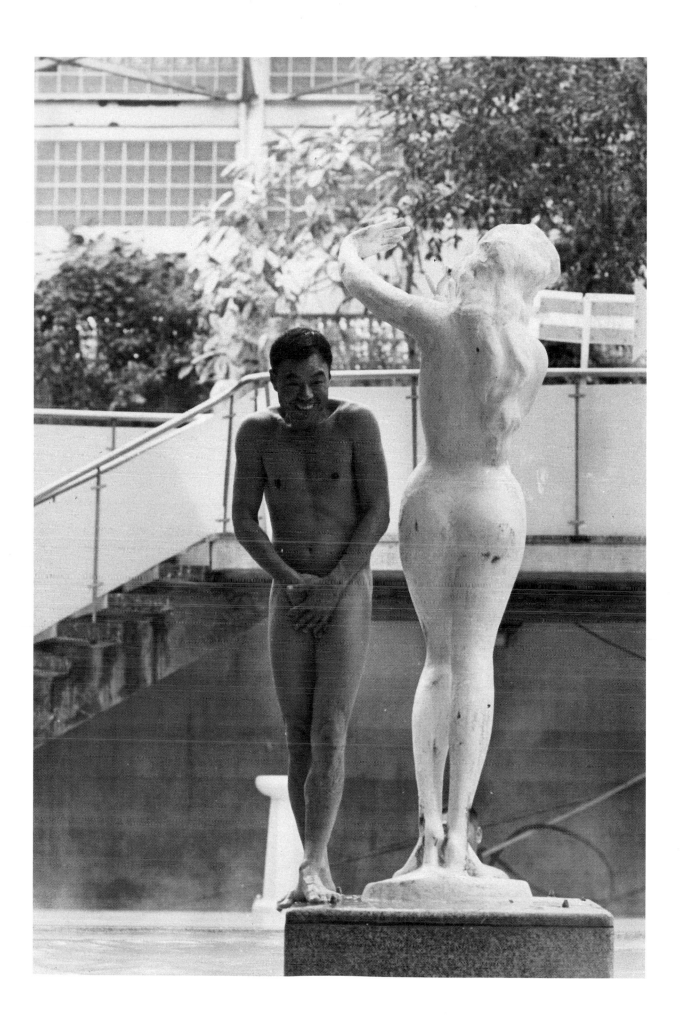

Among the infinite pleasures of
hot-spring bathing are sharing
time with family members, pursu-
ing hobbies, relaxation, and, of
course, bathing.

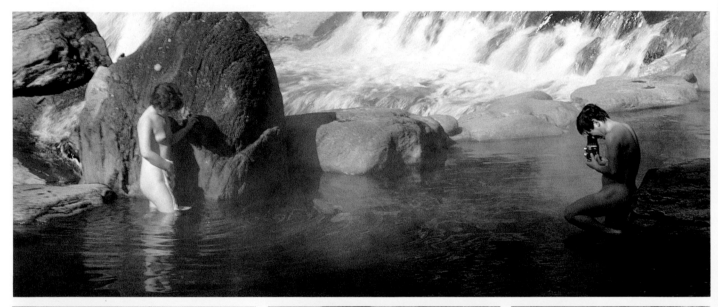

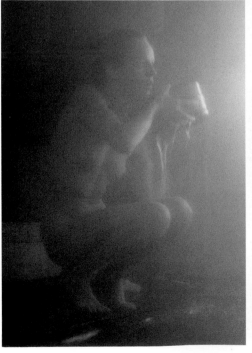

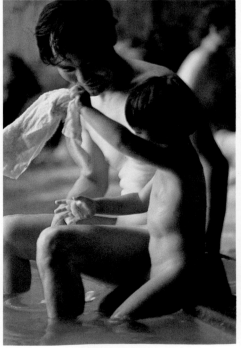

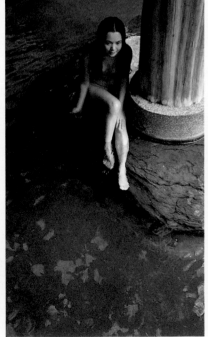

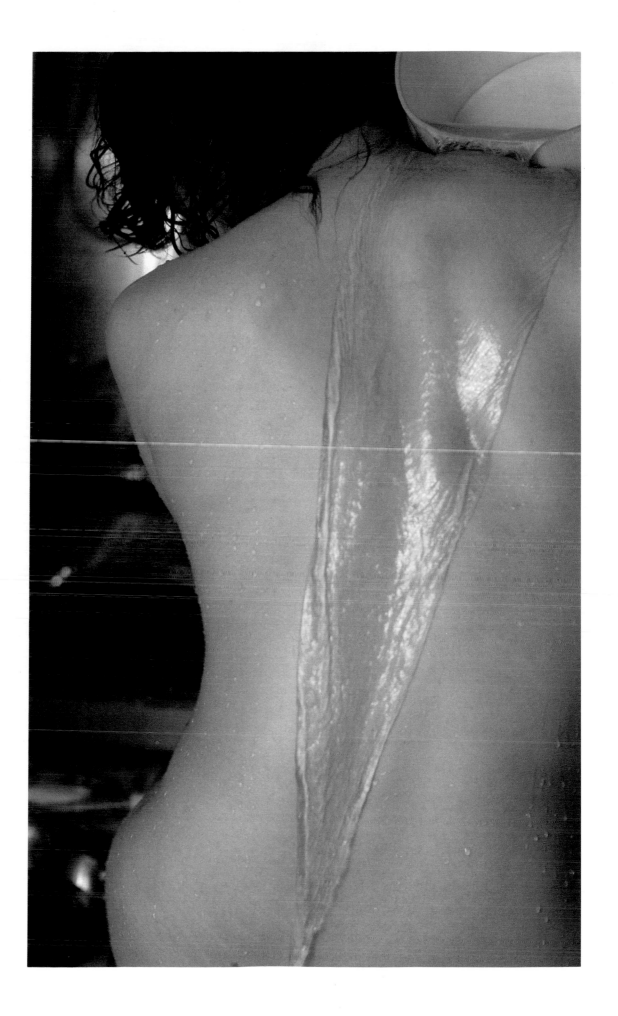

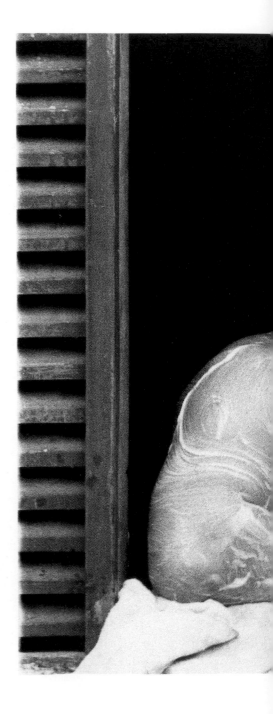

A bath provides refreshing diversion for two young sumo wrestlers after a morning of rigorous training.

Shedding social distinctions along with their clothing, bathers were equal in their common nudity. It would certainly be overstating the case to describe the public bathhouse as an institution of democracy, but it did allow, in a rigidly structured, hierarchical society, a certain easy interaction between people of different classes.

Bathing with others, rather than in solitude, reinforces the most fundamentally cohesive element in Japanese society—the sense of community. Every Japanese individual, as he progresses through the stages of life from infancy to death, projects his familial outlook on all his associations with other people. Life is made up of interlocking circles of *nakama*, emotional fraternities in which he feels comfortable and secure. A legacy no doubt of Japan's agrarian traditions, in which group management of the complicated irrigation systems necessary for successful rice-paddy cultivation required a sharing and collective attitude toward natural resources and human efforts, such group orientations continue to affect all patterns of modern Japanese behavior. Communal bathing is but one example of collective activity that can be seen today in many other realms as well—in patterns of political organization, religious thought, industrial management, education, and even artistic endeavor. To bathe together with one's group—one's friends, colleagues, fellow students, co-workers—is to establish personal bonds and to reaffirm, in the most intimate way, a sense of kinship and interdependence. *Hadaka no tsukiai*—"companions in nudity," or friends who bathe together, the Japanese say, are the closest friends of all. When separated from his *nakama* of the moment, a Japanese feels lost, out of his element, intimidated by alien surroundings. Within his *nakama*, just as when he shares his bath with family or friends, he is warm, secure, and "at home."

In stark contrast, a nervous timidity regarding matters of the human body was characteristic of the Christian culture that spread across Europe following the fall of the Roman Empire. While the Turks elaborated upon Roman bathing practices, Christian Europe retreated further and further from the primitive joy in bathing and human physicality: early Chris-

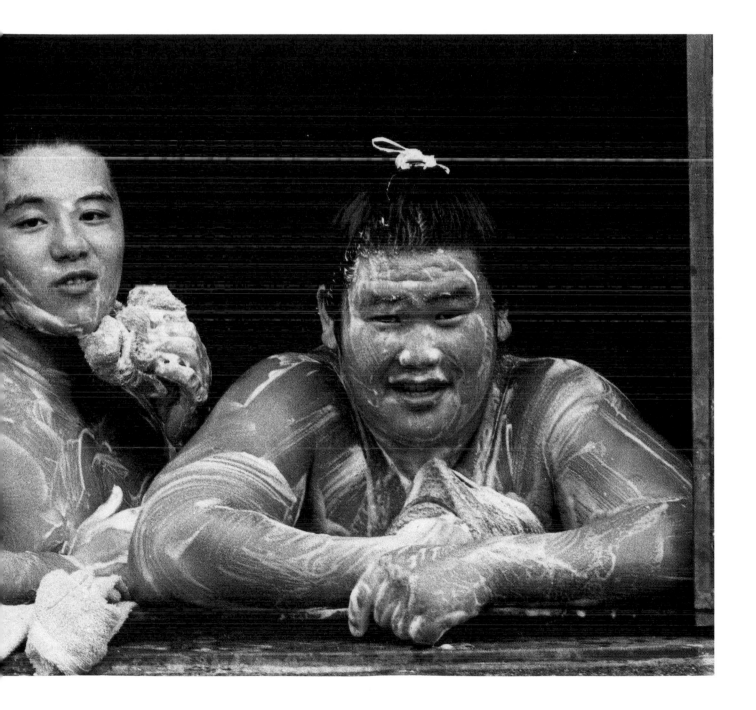

The pleasures of the bath extend over a lifetime. Japanese infants are introduced almost at birth to the physical and spiritual blessings of a long soak in deep hot water with family or friends. (*Lower left photograph courtesy of Norasha*)

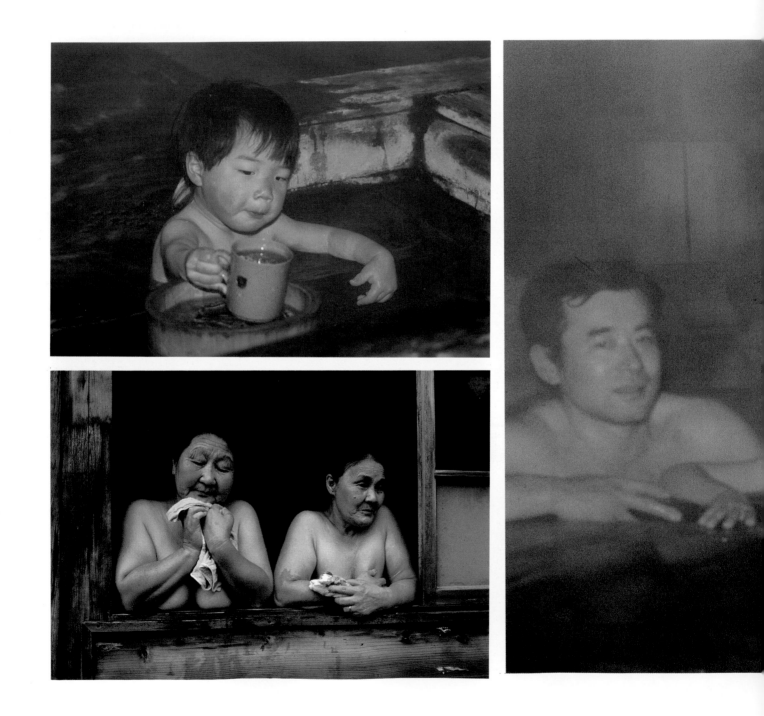

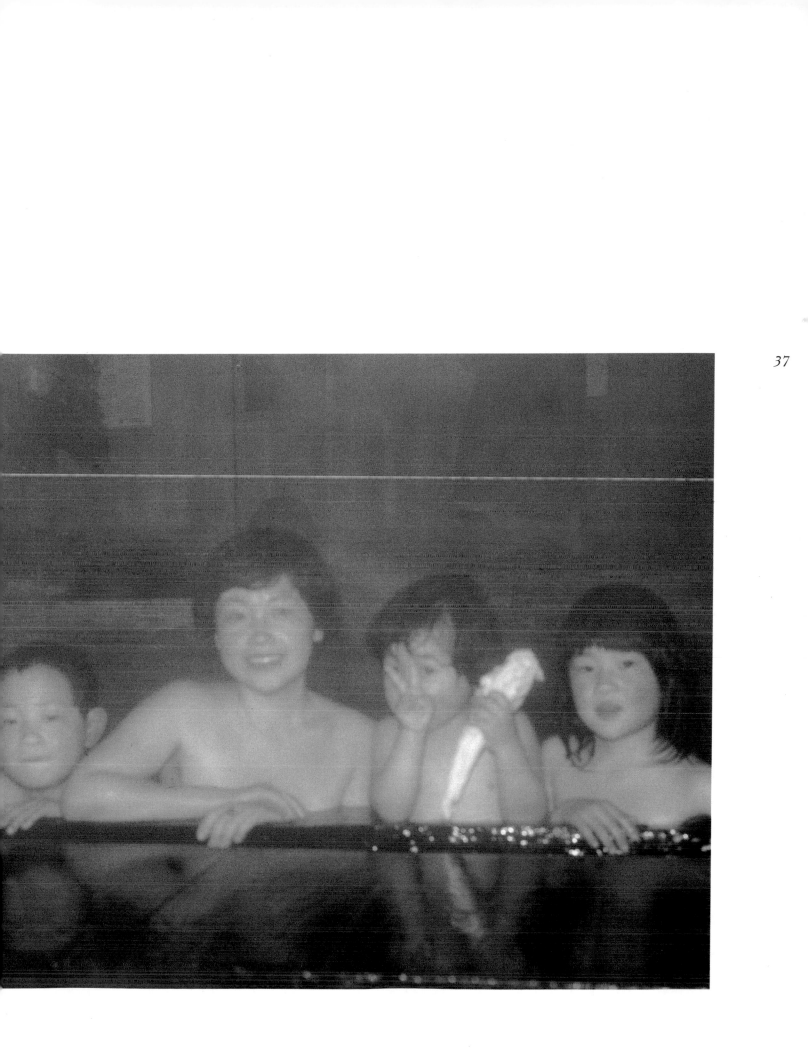

Small or large, rustic or refined, the baths at hot-spring resorts provide a retreat from reality, a misty, warm atmosphere that soothes the body and refreshes the spirit.

tian saints denounced the immorality of communal bathing and public nudity, and some Christian ascetics forbade bathing altogether, regarding filth as a suitable means of mortifying the flesh in penance for sins. Except for a temporary resurgence of communal bathing, a result of Middle Eastern practices influencing the Crusaders, Europe bathed little during the Middle Ages. Elizabeth I of England is said to have behaved rashly in bathing as often as once a month "whether she required it or not." Doctors joined church fathers in condemning bathing as leading toward debauchery and indolence, and it was not until the nineteenth century that modern views of physical hygiene again prescribed regular baths to prevent the spread of disease.

Bathing Japanese-style, whether alone at home or with friends at a public bathhouse or hot spring, is a time of repose and reflection. The surroundings of the bath should be as restful and as close to nature as possible. A bathroom constructed of fine, unvarnished wood and smooth stones that are soft to the touch, illuminated by natural light or by dimly filtered electric light, is preferable, at least in the traditional Japanese aesthetic, to the clinical efficiency of tile and steel and the sterile glare of fluorescent lighting. But if such old-fashioned refinements are seldom possible in an age of plastics, bright colors, and harsh illumination, one can still close one's eyes while sinking deep into the hot water and drift off into a more tranquil frame of mind.

How have the Japanese survived so well the discordant pressures of their modernity? How have they retained, relatively intact, so many of the fundamental values that have strengthened their communal resolve and their sense of identity through the radical changes of circumstance that make up their long history? It is, of course, too much to attribute solely to their baths the success of their cultural continuities. And yet, consider their habit of daily immersion in hot water: the bath instills a feeling of calm, tranquility, and harmony; it refreshes the spirit as it warms and cleans the body; and it does all this across the nation for the majority of the population every day. Perhaps the bath is one of Japan's secret weapons for sur-

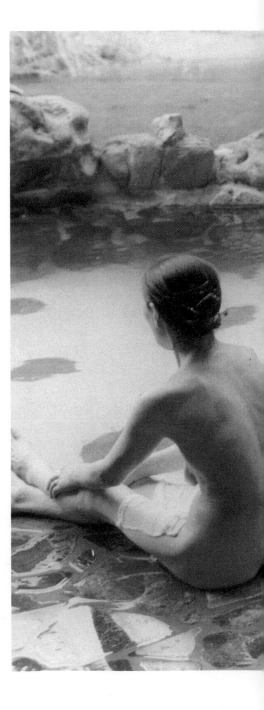

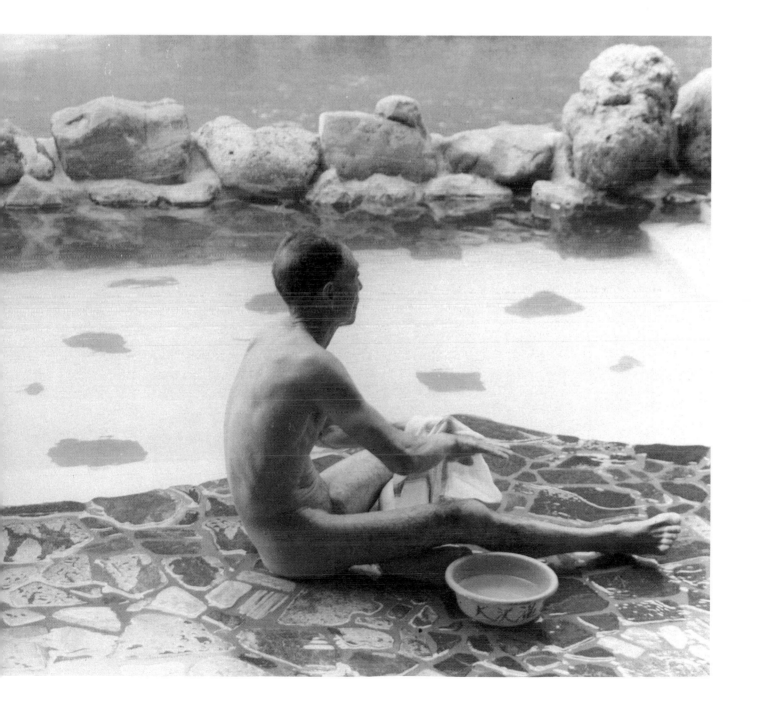

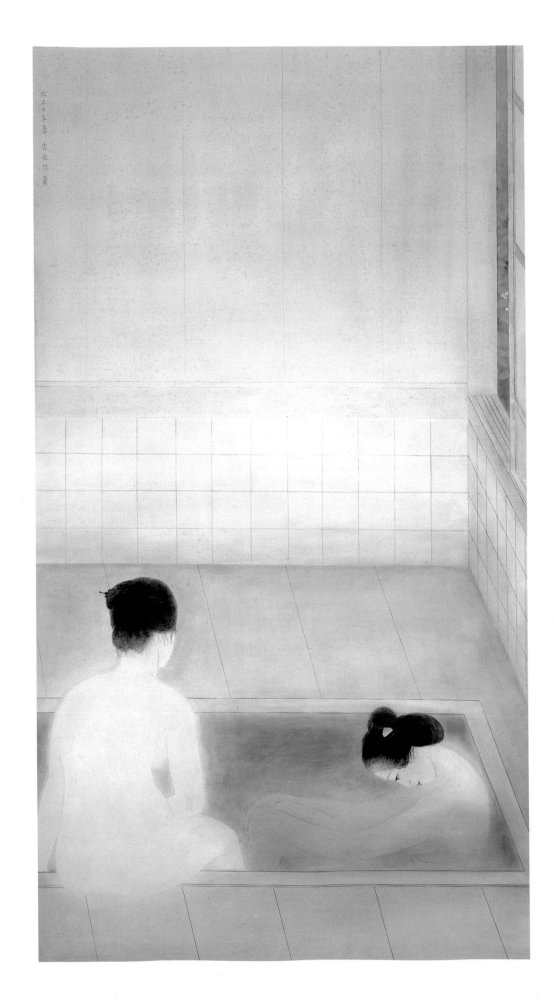

Kokei Kobayashi, *The Hot Spring*, 1918. (*Courtesy of Tokyo National Museum*)

vival in a modern age. Perhaps it is the balm that soothes the aches and bruises brought on by the frenetic pace and conflicting tensions of life as it is everywhere lived today. Perhaps, even, the Japanese bath is a device we all might adopt in surmounting the pressures of our daily lives and in turning back into our selves.

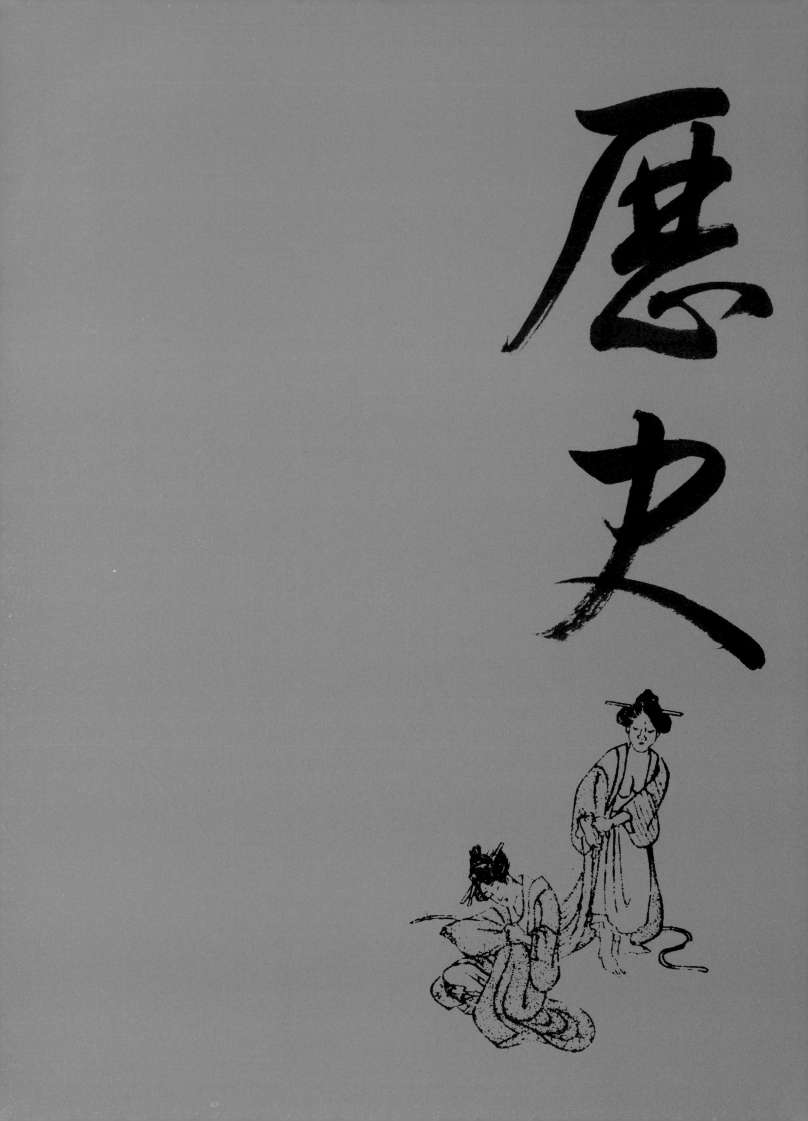

歴史

CHAPTER TWO

The History of Bathing

Who can say, with any certainty, when or where or even how the earliest Japanese took his first bath? *Why* he bathed is far easier to speculate about. He was dirty, there was abundant fresh water available—some of it was even hot since his volcanic environment was lavishly endowed with thermal springs—and he was quick to appreciate the sensual pleasure that cleanliness afforded. Simply put, it felt good to be clean, and in a land with heavy rainfall, streams and rivers everywhere, and plentiful hot and cold natural springs, it was not at all difficult to remain clean.

Little has been recorded of the bathing habits of the early Japanese. The written word came remarkably late in the historical development of the Japanese, and even then, as an unconsolidated tribal people they were less inclined to keep records about their daily life than were their Chinese neighbors on the Asian continent. In seeking information about prehistoric Japan, one must turn to archaeological evidence, to what remains of ancient oral traditions that were collected and written down at a much later date, and to the sketchy accounts of Japan that have been preserved in the dynastic histories of the

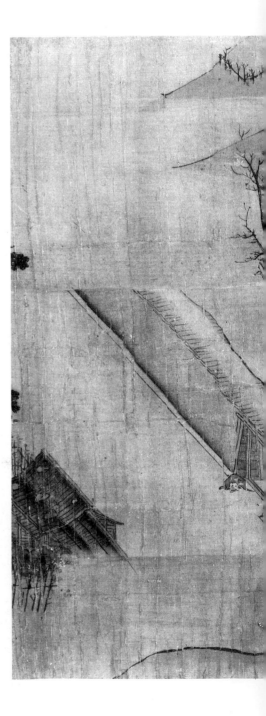

A rustic bathhouse of the Kamakura period. In this illustration from the thirteenth-century narrative scroll *Ippen-shonin Eden*, the itinerant monk Ippen visits one of his spiritual teachers and is immediately offered a bath. Clear cold water is drawn from a well and carried into the adjoining bathhouse, where it is heated in an iron cauldron. (*Courtesy of Kankiko-ji temple; photograph courtesy of Tokyo National Museum*)

44   more literate and more technologically advanced Chinese. In these Chinese histories, references to Japan are generally restricted to chapters devoted to the tributary states of the "Middle Kingdom."

The picture of Japan that emerges, even as early as the third century, is one of a peace-loving and relatively well-ordered society. The Chinese historians, first in the *Wei Chih* (History of the Kingdom of Wei) of A.D. 297 and in subsequent historical records as well, repeatedly noted those aspects of the Japanese "barbarians" to the east that seemed markedly different from Chinese custom: among other things, the Japanese predilection for female rulers, their fondness of strong liquor, and their habits of personal cleanliness. Interpersonal behavior was generally polite, and as part of the rather ceremonial quality that, in the perception of the Chinese, seemed to pervade Japanese life, all religious activities involved some manner of purification or ritual lustration. After Japanese funerals, for example, all members of the family of the deceased were said to join in cleansing themselves in a bath of purification. On dangerous ocean voyages and at other times of social crisis, an individual selected from the group would be forbidden to bathe; it was believed that he would thereby take upon himself any diseases or other pollutants that might imperil the community. If disaster was averted in this way, the individual was rewarded by being allowed to bathe once again; if not, he was killed.

That purity and personal cleanliness were important aspects both of the religious life of the ancient Japanese and of their everyday behavior is further reinforced in the earliest native Japanese attempts to write their own history. The *Kojiki* (Record of Ancient Matters) and the *Nihon Shoki* (Chronicles of Japan), both compiled early in the eighth century, are far less reliable records of historical fact than the Chinese dynastic histories, for they combine legend, mythology, oral traditions, and political propaganda with verifiable events. By inference, however, a careful reading of these pseudohistorical documents offers fascinating insights into the ancient values of the Japanese people. The early Japanese portrayed their gods and many

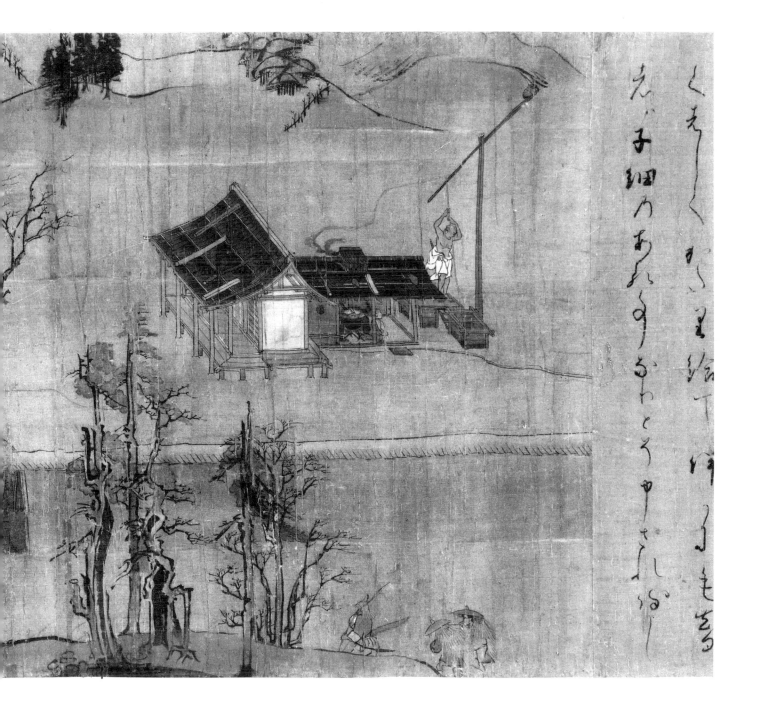

くもゝゝかゝ里絵丁侍子も見

ゑに子細のあるをそのやさしけり

of the spirits of nature in anthropomorphic terms and invested them with the virtues that they cherished themselves. The imperative of personal cleanliness is among their most prominent values. Izanagi, the principal creator-deity, takes a bath on the very first page of the *Kojiki,* and the divine actors of the subsequent myths about the origins of Japan repeatedly immerse themselves in rivers or the sea and engage in all manner of ritualistic purifications. The preface to the *Kojiki* (in the translation of Basil Hall Chamberlain) begins thus:

> Now when chaos had begun to condense, but force and form were not yet manifest, and there was nought named, nought done, who could know its shape? Nevertheless, Heaven and Earth first parted, and the Three Deities performed the commencement of creation; the Passive and Active Essences then developed, and the Two Spirits became the ancestors of all things. Therefore did he [Izanagi] enter obscurity and emerge into light, and the Sun and Moon were revealed by the washing of his eyes; he floated on and plunged into the sea water, and Heavenly and Earthly Deities appeared through the ablutions of his person....

Later in Book I of the *Kojiki,* the same events are depicted in greater detail. Izanami (the female creator-deity) is burned to death in giving birth to the Fire Deity. Izanagi, her spouse, searches for her in Hades, which is described as a foul and polluted place; failing to restore her to life, he returns to the living:

> Therefore, he said, "Nay! Hideous! I have been to a hideous and polluted land. So I will perform the purification of my august person." So he went out to a plain covered with *ahagi* at a small river-mouth near Tachibana in Himuka in the island of Tsukushi, and purified and cleansed himself.

From each of the garments shed by Izanagi before entering this bath was born a new deity, and from the drops of water flowing off his body were born additional gods and goddesses:

> The name of the Deity that was born as he washed his left august eye was Amaterasu-omikami [Heaven-Shining-Great-August-Deity, i.e., the sun]. The name of the Deity that was born as he

washed his right august eye was Tsuki-yomi-no-kami [Moon-Night-Possessor]. The name of the Deity that was next born as he washed his august nose was Take-haya-susa-no-o-no-mikoto [Brave-Swift-Impetuous-Male-Augustness].

The repeated references to bathing in the creation myths and subsequent events of Japanese mythology do not indicate an obsessive or pathological concern with hygiene in the prehistoric Japanese so much as a strong identification of evil and immorality with filth and pollution and—by contrast—of virtue and goodness with cleanliness and purity.

Prayer and purity were closely linked in the ethos of the early Japanese. As in many other primitive societies, frequent ritual lustration and avoidance of pollution were required when communicating with the gods, and elaborate ceremonies were devised to insure the purity of the body as well as the spirit. That cleanliness has survived in Japan as a moral tenet as well as a matter of convenience and comfort may be attributed to the persistence of Shinto attitudes throughout Japanese history. "Religion" is perhaps too weighty a term to use in defining Shinto; it is better described as a loose coalescence of Japanese regional legends, ancestral myths, primitive forms of nature worship, and communal folk beliefs with moral injunctions to maintain harmonious social interactions and ultimately with political attitudes designed to insure the continuity of the state. Central to the Shinto ethos, from the earliest times until the present day, has been its insistence on ritual and actual purity. This "Shinto attitude" is as responsible for the habits of personal hygiene of most Japanese individuals as it is for the fresh, uncluttered aesthetic that pervades Japanese arts, crafts, architecture, cuisine, and virtually all other aspects of traditional Japanese culture.

Japanese do not, of course, think of bathing as a religious act. Nor do they consider their passion for immersing their bodies in the hot water that bubbles forth from natural geothermal springs to be an expression of spirituality. Nevertheless, in the spirit that they bring to bathing there remains a kind of communion with the values and the piety of their forebears.

The first act of a devout worshiper
at a Shinto shrine is to rinse hands
and mouth in a symbolic gesture of
purification.

As Fosco Maraini, with his fine sense of the "interior universe"
of the Japanese, has written:

> The bath is a domestic aspect of ancient purificatory rites, which
> from the earliest times were an essential element of the Shinto
> cult. Now, in the last analysis, every expression of religious feeling
> is a joyful thing; when man feels, however indirectly or remotely
> from his consciousness, that he is in harmony with God, with the
> gods, the invisible, he is happy, at peace with himself and with
> others.

The fact that bathing was practiced in ancient
Japan regularly, frequently, and as an important aspect of everyday social activity is clear. But virtually nothing is known of the
form that bathing took before the sixth or seventh century.
Much, if not all, bathing must have taken place outdoors. The
Japanese myths and Chinese historical records speak only of
ablutions in rivers, ponds, or the sea. The abundance of mineral
springs meant the early Japanese could cleanse and warm their
bodies in pools of hot water wherever it bubbled forth—in river-
beds or from between the rocks of natural geysers. The high
degree of engineering skills required to build the large heated
pools of the Greeks and Romans was rendered unnecessary by
the ready availability of hot-spring water, and consequently such
technology was not developed in Japan until many centuries
after the great bathing emporia of the Roman Empire had
fallen into ruin.

Archaeological studies of prehistoric Japanese
domestic dwellings yield nothing to indicate that large amounts
of water were collected or heated in indoor chambers. The presence of large, sturdy ceramic vessels from early in the first
millennium B.C. suggests that water could be heated in smaller
quantities, and no doubt some of it was used for washing the
body. But for full immersion of the body into water, hot or cold,
the early Japanese still had to go outdoors.

The development of rice cultivation in irrigated
fields during the Yayoi period (200 B.C. to A.D. 250) changed the
patterns of Japanese society in ways that were fundamental and
lasting. While the earlier inhabitants of Japan had lived by hunt-

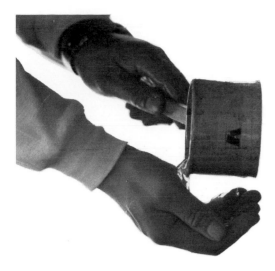

ing and gathering food, the Yayoi people practiced agriculture, which required the establishment of settled, permanent communities. Along with rice cultivation developed the technology for damming streams and controlling the flow of water. This knowledge the Japanese must certainly have applied to their bathing practices as well. Alongside the rivers and hot springs where their ancestors had bathed in free-flowing water, it became possible to build larger bathing pools in which water could be collected and used by entire communities.

Such technology was perfected by the people of the following Tumulus period. Their society consisted of large tribal clans led by powerful families, which in time took on the trappings of a permanent aristocracy. The hierarchy of power that developed through interclan rivalries and warfare ultimately resulted in the pre-eminence of the Yamato clan and, with it, the origins of the Japanese imperial system. In need of symbols of authority to support their rule, the Yamato rulers created the mythology of the imperial lineage descended from the Sun Goddess. It was for this purpose that the quasi-historical *Kojiki* and *Nihon Shoki* were written. Accompanying the establishment of the Yamato rule over subordinate clans was the building of shrine complexes, dedicated to the worship of clan ancestors (real or imagined), and the construction of palaces to house clan rulers and their myriad attendants. The palaces were at the heart of what later came to be Japan's first cities, for surrounding them were increasingly large communities of people gathered to serve the needs of the aristocracy.

Although the scant documentary and archaeological evidence sheds little light on the details of living arrangements, surely the facilities for bathing in these proto-urban centers kept pace with the general advance of technology. Many Shinto shrines that trace their origin to this era, although nominally dedicated to the mythological ancestors of powerful families, were actually established at springs or wells that were critically important to the water supply for an entire community. The rites of *harai* (exorcism and purification) and *misogi* (ritual cleansing) that pervade all aspects of Shinto ceremonies and

Japanese cleansing rituals may be as simple as rinsing one's mouth and hands with a ladle of fresh water at the entrance of a shrine, or as awesome as praying beneath an icy waterfall at a sanctified site deep in the mountains.

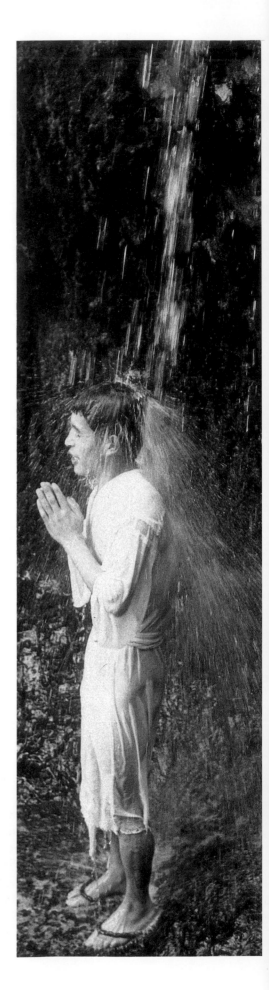

50

that have survived to the present are believed to have been derived from the pragmatic activities of keeping the wells and springs undefiled in order to insure a constant supply of fresh, clean water for drinking, cooking, and bathing.

Devotional practices at Shinto shrines today continue to echo the imperatives of cleanliness and purity that stem from these archaic origins. Devout worshipers approaching a shrine today stop first at a fountain in its outer precincts to rinse their hands and mouths in a symbolic gesture of purification. This is one example of *misogi,* as is the practice of young men bathing at night in cold rivers or standing in prayer beneath freezing waterfalls to cleanse the soul and strengthen the spirit before attacking some particularly challenging task. The blessing of purification *(harai)* conferred by Shinto priests on worshipers may be either a simple gesture of waving a sacred branch over their heads or, at its most elaborate, it may take the form of extended ceremonies and prayers by the emperor and Shinto priests for the purification and welfare of the nation as a whole.

Shintoism was not the only religion that yielded a profound effect on Japanese society and its attitudes toward bathing. The arrival of Buddhism in Japan in the middle of the sixth century launched an era of cultural transformation that was not to be equaled in extent until the "modernization" of Japanese society during the Meiji era thirteen hundred years later. Buddhism, recommended to the Japanese ruler by the king of Paekche, one of the three early Korean kingdoms, quickly overcame the resistance of traditionalist factions at the Japanese court and within a century was embraced by nearly the entire aristocracy. But acceptance of the continental religion entailed far more than conversion to a new faith: accompanying Buddhism came nearly every aspect of the civilization of China, which in turn had its sources in societies covering the entire continent of Asia and the Middle East.

The Japanese, still relatively backward in their level of cultural development, were understandably dazzled by the splendors of continental culture and, under the enlightened leadership of such political figures as the regent Shotoku, were quick to adopt its physical attributes along with its spiritual values. Virtually nothing was left untouched by influence from China: social and political organization, education, food, dress, architecture, and other aspects of Japanese life and work. While the cultural imports took hold most dramatically at the court in the Yamato Plain and in the few other centers of population, they soon spread throughout Japan, thanks to an extensive program of political unification. This attempt at national consolidation was carried out, in large part, through the development of a system of regional Buddhist temples controlled by the imperial court.

The thoroughgoing program of social, political, cultural, and technological modernization launched by conversion to the new religion proceeded rapidly. In 552, the date generally given for the first introduction of Buddhist imagery and theological texts from Korea, Japan was still a land of loosely organized tribes, struggling with one another for political hegemony over a society that was culturally and technologically far less advanced than its continental neighbors. Within a mere two centuries of that date, Japan had a political system centralized in a well-educated urban bureaucracy at the city of Nara, itself a new city laid out on an up-to-date Chinese plan; a highly cultured aristocracy was supported by the output of great agricultural estates; Buddhism was recognized as the national religion; and the Japanese countryside was being altered by a zeal for construction that was everywhere creating new cities, palaces, and temples.

The success of Buddhism—and, indeed, the success of the entire cultural transformation that had followed the introduction of the new religion—was celebrated in 753 by an event of notable significance. That year Emperor Shomu led the ceremonies at Nara dedicating a great gilded bronze image of the Buddha at a new temple adjoining the imperial court. The new technological and cultural sophistication of the Japanese people was manifest in the huge statue, for its construction drew not only on the resources of the entire nation but also on the support of all of Buddhist Asia. Gifts offered to the great Buddha came from as far away as Persia, and around the statue was built the Todai-ji temple, the keystone in the national network of Buddhist institutions that linked the far-flung provinces to the imperial court.

Among the many subordinate buildings surrounding the Great Buddha Hall at the Todai-ji temple was the Nigatsu-do (Second-Month Hall), a religious structure that symbolizes the fusion of Buddhist ritual with the native Japanese passion for cleanliness. Built over the principal spring providing water to the temple, the Nigatsu-do was the site of the *mizutori* rite, a ceremonial drawing of water for purifying the Buddha, which took place each year during the second month of the lunar calendar. The Nigatsu-do also served as a bathhouse for the monks residing at Todai-ji, and in time its large bath was also made available, as a charitable public service, to the nonclerical community as well.

While the Buddhist sutras, from their origins in India, made frequent mention of the virtues of cleanliness and the spiritual merit gained by the historical Buddha and his disciples from bathing the poor and the diseased, this association of bathing with public charity retained little more than its symbolic meaning in China and Korea. In Japan, however, it harmonized well with the native enthusiasm for cleanliness and was given literal application. Most other temples in the capital city of Nara, and in the provinces as well, possessed a large bathhouse whose use by commoners helped promote the religion's reputation for compassion and benevolence among the Japanese people.

While none of the original bathhouses of the Nara period remains, temple documents of the time preserve a good deal of information about them. Construction records at the Horyu-ji temple, for example, provide details of a new bathhouse built there in 747 that contained a copper tub nearly five feet in diameter and four feet deep. At the Daian-ji temple an even larger tub was built not long afterward. These copper tubs were used for heating large quantities of water, which was then drawn off by pipes or buckets and used in smaller wooden vats

Scale drawings of the Nigatsu-do at the Todai-ji temple in Nara. Built over a spring that was the principal source of water for the great religious complex, this hall also served as bathhouse for the monks and congregation of Todai-ji. In the center of the building is the huge metal cauldron in which bath water was heated. (*Courtesy of Agency for Cultural Affairs, Japan*)

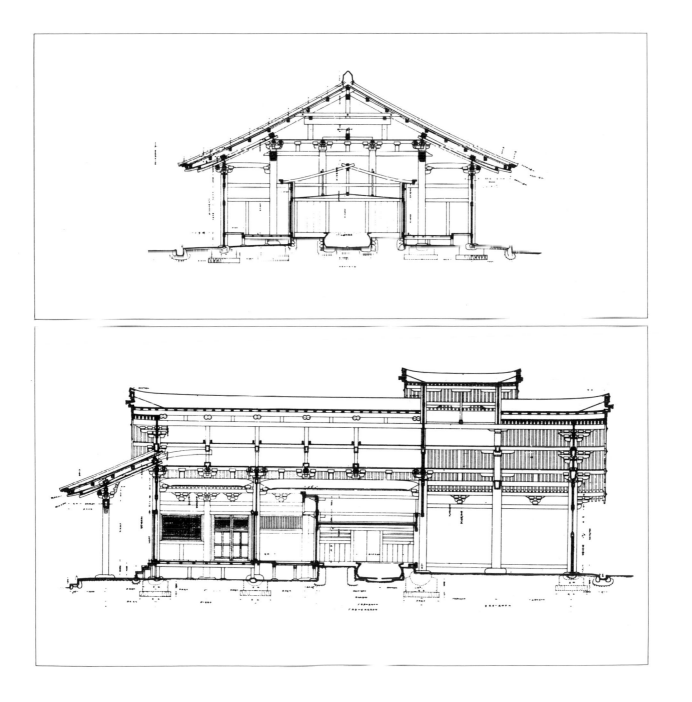

Bathing, faith, and healing merge at the Imagami hot spring, deep in the mountains of Yamagata Prefecture. For more than a thousand years, the waters of Imagami have been considered a potent cure for leprosy and other dread skin diseases. The single bathhouse there has become a shrine to the healing deity Imagami Sanjo Daigongen; worshipers immerse themselves in the waters and pray for as long as six or seven hours a day. (*Courtesy of Norasha*)

by monks and laymen. The large metal cauldrons were counted among the chief assets of a temple, and during periods of fierce rivalry between religious sects the tubs were often stolen from one temple and installed in another. In the year 1199, for example, monks from the Kofuku-ji temple in Nara raided Horyu-ji, destroying some of the sacred statuary and stealing the tub from the temple bathhouse. In most of the bathhouses, there was a shrine to the deity of the bath, and it was the custom to wash the statue on certain ceremonial occasions.

At first it was the temples themselves that attracted converts or faithful worshipers by providing baths as a social service. In time, however, it came to be a religious custom for wealthy patrons of a temple to sponsor baths for the poor. Known as *seyoku,* this practice of "charitable baths" grew more widespread as Buddhism developed from a purely monastic religion to a popular faith with large congregations of lay worshipers. Comparable to the Roman Catholic practice of making cash contributions to a church so that special masses might be offered in the name of a beloved family member, in Japan *seyoku* could be arranged at a temple by donating money or large quantities of firewood or fuel for heating the bath water. A single bath might be donated or, in the case of large contributions, charity baths might be arranged in perpetuity. Through this means, wealthy believers might gain religious merit during their lifetimes and even attempt to secure the repose of their souls after death.

One of the most renowned paragons of Buddhist charity in Japanese history is Empress Komyo, consort of Emperor Shomu. It was Shomu who had decreed the construction of the Great Buddha and the Todai-ji temple and who was most responsible for the spread of Buddhism to all provinces by the end of the eighth century. Celebrated as much for her piety as for her great beauty, Empress Komyo is said to have vowed to bathe one thousand beggars with her own hands in the bathhouse of the Hokke-ji temple at Nara. This she proceeded to do. Legend has it that after scrubbing nine hundred and ninety-nine beggars, she looked up to see that the last was a leper. The

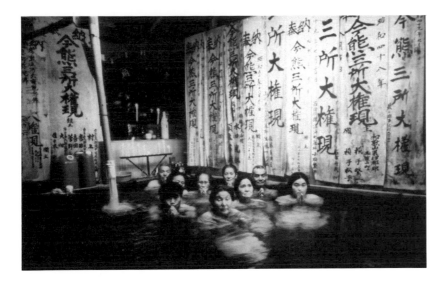

virtuous empress did not flinch from her task, however, and the thousandth beggar revealed himself to her as the Buddha, who had come to aid her progress toward enlightenment.

The association between bathing and Buddhism is further elucidated in the *Samboe,* a collection of Buddhist fables and tales compiled in 984 by the scholarly courtier Minamoto no Tamenori for the edification of Imperial Princess Sonshi shortly after she had left the court to become a nun. One section of the *Samboe* is devoted to the bathing practices of Buddhist monks, as inspired by the saintly example of Sakyamuni and his disciples:

> On the fourteenth and twenty-ninth days of each month, a great bath is prepared in every temple and all the monks bathe. This is because the Convocation is held on the following day. The bath is also prepared on many other unspecified days, in accordance with the need of individual monks.
>
> In the *Sutra on Baths and Bathing for the Clergy* it is said: "The Elder Jivaka, son of Amrapali, had an idea one night as he was falling asleep, and the next morning he went to the Buddha and said, 'I have busied myself with worldly affairs, and have not yet earned merit. Now I would like to invite the Buddha and his disciples to wash themselves in the bath I have prepared. I pray that all sentient beings may be cleansed of the worldly filth of ignorance.'
>
> "The Buddha said, 'Very good! There is no measure of the merit in this. For priestly bathing, seven objects are used in the bath room. There are seven salutary effects of bathing, and seven benefits accrue. The seven objects are firewood, pure water, bean husks for scrubbing, bath oil to moisten, cool and soften the body, finely ground ashes, willow-twig toothpicks and bath robes. The seven salutary effects of bathing are relaxation of the body; avoidance of colds; avoidance of pains; avoidance of chills; avoidance of fever; avoidance of filth; and refreshing of the body and clearing of vision. As for the seven benefits, the first is that disorders of the Four Elements are prevented, and in every life into which you are reborn you will be lovely in form and pure in person. Second, filth is washed away from the place where it lodges and pollutes. Third, the body is always kept fragrant, and one's garments remain clean and fresh. Fourth, the skin of the body is

The water of Japanese hot springs heals, refreshes, and at times even massages. At Kita in Tochigi Prefecture, a hot-spring waterfall pounds the aching muscles of bathers, leaving them relaxed and invigorated. (*Courtesy of Norasha*)

made soft, smooth and lustrous, as it can be made by nothing else. Fifth, many persons will follow and serve you, and brush away the dust and sweep away the filth from your path. Sixth, the odor of the mouth is fragrant and clean, and the words you speak will be followed by the people. Seventh, at birth you will be naturally clothed and adorned with everlastingly brilliant jewels. Indeed, those who are born into this world with pleasant features admired by others, and who are pure and clean and lustrous-skinned, are those who, in their former lives, provided baths for monks and have been thus rewarded. These rewards are also obtained as the result of providing baths for monks: birth as the son of a great minister, and enjoyment of a wealth of treasures; birth in the house of a great king, where you are bathed with fragrant incense and perfumed water; protection in all four directions through the power of the Four Celestial Kings; illumination of the darkness of night by the sun, moon and the constellations; and adornment with the Seven Jewels of Indra, enjoyment of a long life, reaching the world beyond the Four Seas ruled by the Great Kings, where you may revel in many pleasures and have a fragrant body, and revel in the pleasures of the Six Desire Heavens to the utmost, and dwell in the perfect quiescent state in Brahma's Heaven.'"

Clearly, the donating of baths to the clergy and to the poor was well worth the expense to any aristocrat or wealthy person able to afford it.

The lore of Buddhist "saints" of later eras frequently includes charitable acts relating to providing baths for the faithful or the needy. Kobo Daishi (774–835), founder of the Shingon sect and perhaps the most revered religious teacher in Japanese history, traveled widely throughout the country, preaching, undergoing religious austerities, and working miracles of faith everywhere he went. Many regional legends name him as the creator of local hot springs: most often he would arrive at a town whose inhabitants were suffering from disease and, striking his staff upon a rock, would bring forth plentiful hot water to cure their ills. Other tales of Kobo Daishi's prowess describe his ability to withstand harsh physical austerities. From his example, later monks and priests of the esoteric sects of Buddhism bathed in the wintry sea or stood under icy waterfalls as

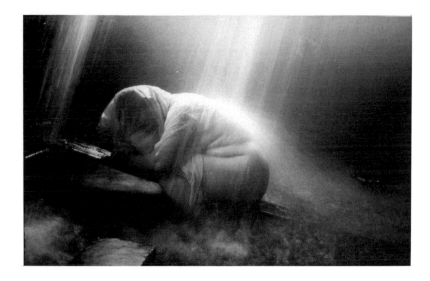

means to strengthen their religious concentration or to fortify themselves for difficult undertakings.

Another holy man who played a memorable role in the history of bathing was the monk Chogen (1121–1206), one of Kobo Daishi's most beloved successors. Chogen was renowned as an engineer, inventor, and builder of huge religious projects: It was Chogen who was given the imperial commission to rebuild the Great Buddha Hall at the Todai-ji temple after it was burned in 1180. It was he who tirelessly collected funds throughout Japan for this enormous construction project, and it was also he who devised new engineering techniques to transport the equipment and huge wooden pillars used in rebuilding the temple. But the Japanese remember Chogen most as a builder of bathhouses. Early in his career, recognizing the need for larger baths at temples for serving the masses, he began assembling construction brigades to build bathhouses at temples all over the country. Chogen's public-works schemes also inspired the wealthy to contribute funds or fuel for temples' charity baths.

Until the establishment of public baths in the sixteenth and seventeenth centuries, it was chiefly Buddhist temples that provided bathing facilities for the Japanese populace. The aristocracy and the powerful military families had private baths in their palaces and castles, but it was the responsibility of the Buddhist clergy to bathe the people at large. The charity baths played so important a role in the social activity of Japanese Buddhist temples that Chinese and Korean monks visiting Japan in later centuries frequently remarked on the practice and recommended that it be reintroduced to the temples in their native lands.

Although the elegant life of the Japanese aristocracy has been described in meticulous detail in the diaries of court ladies and in superb works of fiction written during the Heian and Fujiwara periods (eighth to twelfth centuries) when the aristocratic culture was at its peak, these writings are surprisingly reticent on the subject of the bath. Perhaps bathing was so taken for granted that it was thought unworthy of comment, or

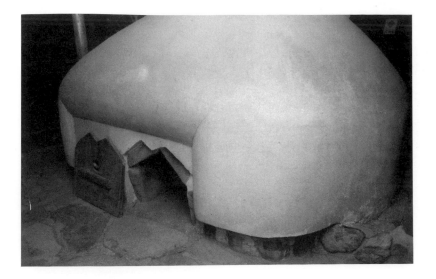

One of the most ancient forms of bathing in Japan is the *kama-buro* or "kiln bath." Adjoining a fire chamber, where water is boiled, is a tightly sealed steam room with thick clay walls. Once common, today *kama-buro* are patronized by people seeking novel bathing experiences and can be found only at Yase, near Kyoto, and a few other sites.

perhaps the act of washing the body was deemed too inelegant a subject for detailed description. Whatever the reason, though a very great deal is known about the dress and amusements, love affairs and ceremonies, superstitions and religious beliefs of the court aristocracy, relatively little information on their bathing habits is to be found. The fact that they bathed is clear. Unlike their latter-day counterparts at the European courts of Elizabeth I of England or Louis XIV of Versailles, who were equally cultivated in matters of dress, literary pursuits, and political intrigue but thoroughly negligent of personal hygiene, the noblemen and ladies at the imperial Heian court in Kyoto continued to uphold the standards of cleanliness of their supposedly divine ancestors. In the language of their gracious lives, the words for good, beautiful, and clean were closely related, and insofar as the nobility noticed the common people at all they were considered dirty, vulgar, and ugly.

The early court diaries, novels, and essays do mention visits to hot springs, as well as private baths at the court, but they do not dwell on the details of bathing or the technology for providing quantities of hot water to the large population inhabiting Kyoto's palaces. Even the inquiring eye and writing-brush of Sei Shonagon (b. 965?), author of *The Pillow Book*, made little note of baths. In her compendium of court gossip and sharp observations of the manners and idiosyncracies of her contemporaries, she remarks on the care entailed in presenting a properly clean and attractive appearance but says little about how it was done. In her listing of Things That Make One's Heart Beat Faster, she includes: "To wash one's hair, make one's toilet, and put on scented robes, even if not a soul sees one, these preparations still produce an inner pleasure." And among her Depressing Things: "To take a hot bath when one has just woken is not only depressing; it actually puts one in a bad humor." Although Sei Shonagon clearly preferred her baths at night, it was important that people washed in the morning; among her listing of Things That Give an Unclean Feeling, she counts "someone who is late in washing his hands in the morning." On the other hand, she preferred amorous young men of

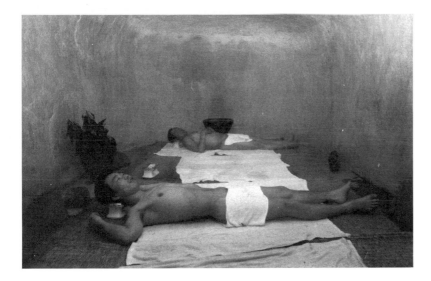

the court to be rather leisurely about their morning washing,
attending first to their love poems and other affairs of the heart:

A young bachelor of an adventurous nature comes home at
dawn, having spent the night in some amorous encounter.
Though he still looks sleepy, he immediately draws his inkstone
to him and, after carefully rubbing it with ink, starts to write his
next-morning letter. He does not let his brush run down the paper in a careless scrawl, but puts himself heart and soul into the
calligraphy. What a charming figure he makes as he sits there by
himself in an easy posture, with his robe falling slightly open! It is
a plain, unlined robe of pure white, and over it he wears a cloak
of rose-yellow or crimson. As he finishes his letter, he notices that
the white robe is still damp from the dew, and for a while he gazes
at it fondly.

Then he makes arrangements for delivering the letter. Instead of calling one of the ladies in attendance, he takes the trou-
ble to get up and select a page-boy who seems suitable for the
task. Summoning the boy to his side, he whispers his instructions
and hands over the letter. The page leaves for the lady's house,
and for some time the gentleman watches him disappear in the
distance. As he sits there, he quietly murmurs some appropriate
passage from the sutras.

Now one of his servants comes to announce that his wash-
ing-water and morning gruel have been prepared in the neigh-
boring wing. The gentleman goes there, and soon he is leaning
against the reading-desk and looking at some Chinese poems,
from which he now and then reads out a passage that he has particularly enjoyed—altogether a charming sight!

Presently he performs his ablutions and changes into a
white court cloak, which he wears without any trousers. Thus at-
tired, he starts reciting the sixth scroll of the Lotus Sutra from
memory. A pious gentleman indeed—or so one might think,
except that at just this moment the messenger returns (he cannot
have had far to go) and nods encouragingly to his master, who
thereupon instantly interrupts his recitation and, with what
might strike one as sinful haste, transfers his attention to the
lady's reply.

All of court life was imbued with a ritualistic
orderliness decreed in part by a complex system of taboos, su-

Detail from a seventeenth-century screen entitled *Entertainments at a House of Pleasure*. During the Edo period, lavish brothels and tea-houses usually provided bath-houses where guests could relax and refresh themselves. Here a patron is seen disappearing into the steam room, attended by young women called *yuna*. (*Courtesy of Suntory Museum of Art*)

perstitious prescriptions, and semireligious requirements and prohibitions. One could not travel in certain directions, for example, if the calendar deemed them unlucky that day. One was forbidden from appearing at court or engaging in certain rituals immediately after suffering an illness or other inauspicious defilement. Similarly, bathing was regulated by the calendar. In a collection of pronouncements set down to guide his descendants on proper behavior, the nobleman Fujiwara no Morosuke (908–60) writes: "Choose an auspicious day for your bath; bathe once every five days." Except for the case of newborn babies, in need of more frequent baths, or patients who went to hot springs for medical treatment (among other spas, *The Pillow Book* and *The Tale of Genji* recommend the waters of Arima, Iyo, and Tamatsukuri as particularly efficacious), the Japanese practice of daily bathing was not to become commonplace until a later era.

Despite their general diligence in adhering to the superstitious notions that regulated their lives, Heian courtiers seem to have, on occasion, ignored the taboos when considerations of personal cleanliness so demanded. For example, in his diary entry for the first day of the fifth month in the year 1009, Fujiwara no Yukinari writes:

> Although some have said that one should not wash hair in the fifth month and that it is forbidden to bathe on the first day of any month, I consulted the almanac, and seeing not only that it was good to wash one's hair on the first day of the fifth month but also that bathing on this day would even bring long life and good fortune; however, in order to achieve great happiness I should not go out for three days. So, therefore, I bathed and washed my hair this morning.

Similarly, in the diary of the great court poet Fujiwara no Teika the entry for the thirtieth day of the fourth month of the year 1200 reads:

> Even though it was strongly admonished that one not bathe on this day to avoid plagues, diseases, and various other misfortunes, because I was feeling unclean I decided to bathe anyway.

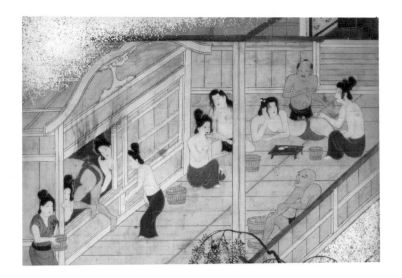

The association of calendrical superstitions with bathing practices persisted, despite such occasional infractions, until well into the Edo period (1603–1868), and on inauspicious days the public bathhouses of that era were often nearly empty.

       One of the most glorious series of ceremonies at the Heian court was that celebrating the birth of an imperial prince. Elaborate washing rituals, comparable in significance to the baptismal rites of Christianity, followed the birth of any Japanese child; as might be expected, those lavished on a child of imperial birth were of special splendor. *The Tale of Genji* and other contemporary works of romantic fiction describe the natal baths of infant princes, many of such passages inspired no doubt by the celebrations that followed the birth in 1008 of Prince Atsuhira to Lady Shoshi, consort of Emperor Ichijo. Shoshi was the daughter of Fujiwara no Michinaga (966–1027), the prime minister and most influential figure at court; the birth of his grandson, the crown prince, was the ultimate confirmation of Michinaga's power and was consequently an event calling for extraordinary celebration. Page after page of the diary of Murasaki Shikibu (978–1016), author of *The Tale of Genji* and one of Lady Shoshi's principal attendants, is devoted to the ceremonies that surrounded the week of twice-daily baths of the infant prince. Murasaki describes not only the preparation of the tubs and utensils used for the prince and the ritualistic drawing of specially purified waters, but also every detail of the finery worn by the attendants (virtually all members of the highest ranks of the aristocracy were present), the elaborate meals served, the gifts presented, and the poems and prayers recited. What follows is an excerpt from her diary entry for the eleventh day of the ninth month of the year 1008. The ceremonials described in entries for successive days became, if possible, even more elaborate:

> The first bath must have taken place at about six in the evening. The torches were lit and Her Majesty's servants carried in the hot water. They were wearing white vestments over their short green robes, and both the tubs and the stands were covered in white cloth. Chikamitsu, Chief of the Weaving Office, and Chief At-

62

tendant Nakanobu bore the tubs up to the blinds and passed
them in to the two women in charge of the water, Kiyoiko no
Myobu and Harima, who in turn made sure it was only lukewarm. Then two other women, Omoku and Muma, poured it
into sixteen pitchers and emptied what remained into the bath
tub. They were all wearing gauze mantles, with trains and jackets
of taffeta, and had their hair done up with hairpins and white rib-
bons; it looked most attractive.

Lady Saisho was in charge of the bathing and Lady Dai-
nagon acted as her assistant; both were wearing aprons which
were most unusual and very elegant.

His Excellency carried the baby Prince in his arms, Lady
Koshosho with the sword and Miya no Naishi with the tiger's
head leading the way. Miya no Naishi's jacket had a pine-cone
pattern and her train had a wave design woven into it, giving it
the appearance of a printed seascape. The waistband was of thin
gauze embroidered with a Chinese vine pattern. Lady Koshosho's train was decorated with autumn grasses, butterflies, and
birds sketched in glittering silver. No one was free to do exactly
as they pleased because there was a limit to what could be done
with the material so she had obviously tried something unusual
at the waistline.

His Excellency's two sons Yorimichi and Norimichi, Minor
Captain Minamoto no Masamichi, and various others scattered
rice with great shouts, seeing who could make the most noise.
The Bishop of the Jodo-ji, who was there in the capacity of religious protector, had to cover his head and face with a fan for fear
of being hit; the younger women were greatly amused.

The Doctor of Letters, who read out the text from the
Classics, was Fifth Secretary Hironari. He stood below the bal-
ustrade and read out the opening passage from the *Records of the
Grand Historian*, while behind him twenty men, ten of Fifth and
ten of Sixth Rank, stood in two lines twanging their bows.

The baths at court and in the residential palaces
of the nobility seem to have been of rather simple construction.
Deep tubs in which the entire body might be immersed in hot
water were relatively rare except at hot-spring resorts, where
natural hot water gushed forth from the earth at no cost to anyone. Elsewhere, where water had to be heated and consequently

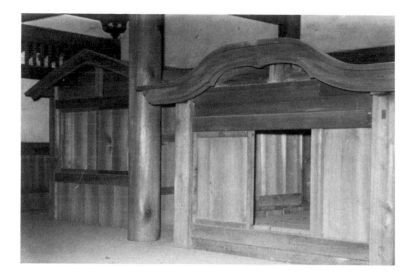

was in relatively short supply, baths took the form of a sudatorium, or steam bath. The bathing chamber was built over a
firebox, which when stoked with burning wood heated both the
air in the room and a tub of water; the boiling water gave off
steam, which filled the small room. The bather would sit in this
wet steam-room, his perspiration cleansing his body. Soap was
not used in Japan until the nineteenth century; instead, the
body was scrubbed with various herbs, with the *hechima* gourd
(luffa), or with bags filled with rice bran. To conclude a bath, hot
or lukewarm water was splashed over the body to rinse it clean.
The wooden floor of the room was fitted with drains so that
dirty water could be rinsed away easily and would not collect on
the floor. Although tubs in which the entire body could be
soaked were not unknown, they were relatively rare before the
sixteenth century.

The latter half of the twelfth century witnessed
the clash of a number of warrior families vying with one another
for the privilege of "protecting" the emperor but actually struggling to dominate the imperial court and to assert their inde-
pendent power. For the next seven hundred years, although the
aristocratic court remained in Kyoto and the emperor retained
nominal authority over the country, the actual locus of power
shifted from one military house to another. The most powerful
clan at any given time was headed by a warlord who took the
ancient title of shogun, swearing to protect and preserve the im
perial family and to wield power only in the name of the emperor. Under first the Minamoto shoguns, who established their
power base at Kamakura, then the Ashikaga shoguns, who returned the military court to Kyoto, and finally the Tokugawa
family and its long-lived shogunate at Edo (present-day Tokyo),
the real governance of Japan was transferred from the imperial
court to a feudalistic system in which power was based on prowess in battle and on an increasingly complex hierarchy of feudal
loyalties.

Since power in a military society was deter-
mined not by family name or ancient lineage but rather by the
number of allies loyal to one's cause and the number of warriors

This painted wooden *ema* of a blissful child in a bath is a votive offering, probably presented to a shrine by a troubled mother whose child resisted bathing. (*Courtesy of Shigemasa Kishi Collection, Osaka*)

one could marshal on the battlefield, the period following the decline of the imperial court was marked by civil disorder, decentralization, and bloody warfare. A samurai's virtue was measured not by his literary skill, his scholarly erudition, or his amorous exploits but rather by the strength of his loyalty to an overlord or his readiness to die in battle. Instead of the courtly arts of music and calligraphy long cherished by his aristocratic predecessors, the feudal samurai cultivated strength of body and spirit.

In the atmosphere of austerity and discipline that characterized military life, it is not surprising that pleasures of the flesh and comforts of the body should have played a lesser role in the samurai code of *bushido* ("the way of the warrior"). Cleanliness and purity were valued by the samurai only insofar as they reinforced his spiritual concentration and the single-minded purposefulness with which he strengthened his mind and body. The rules of behavior passed on from generation to generation in a samurai household required that personal cleanliness be maintained if it could be done frugally and without unnecessary concessions to personal comfort. Bathing could be accomplished in cold water as well as hot, and often was. Indeed, subjecting the body to cold water was seen as a means of fortifying the spirit. Following the example of earlier religious ascetics, the samurai practiced bathing in cold rivers or meditating under icy waterfalls. *The Tale of the Heike,* the great twelfth-century saga depicting the rivalry of the Heike and Minamoto clans, provides several illustrations of samurai austerities. In one such passage, a warrior named Mongaku, determined to renounce the life of battle for the priesthood, makes a pilgrimage to famous religious sites:

> He went to Kumano and decided to seclude himself at Nachi. For the first step of his austerities he went down to the basin of the Nachi waterfall, determined to bathe in the water. It was toward the middle of the twelfth month when he arrived there. Deep snow lay upon the ground, and icicles hung thickly from the trees. The stream in the ravine was silent. Freezing blasts swept down from the mountain tops. The waterfall's white threads

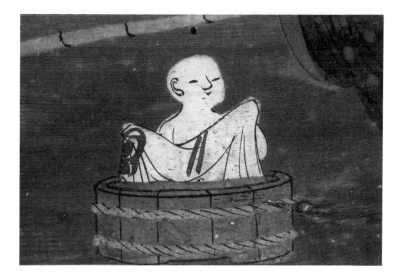

were frozen into crystalline clusters, and the trees were wrapped in white. Mongaku did not hesitate for an instant; he went down to the pool and waded in until the water reached his neck. Then he began to intone an invocation to Fudo-myo-o in Sanskrit.

More conventional and more comfortable forms of bathing were available to samurai society, of course, and were not neglected. But in military romances like *The Tale of the Heike,* the pleasures of bathing in hot water are given a softer, more feminine tone than the descriptions of such heroic austerities as Mongaku's. In another passage, the *Heike* describes a different type of bath. Shigehira, a great Heike general, has been shamed by being captured in battle (rather than dying by his own sword) and has been sent in disgrace as a prisoner to the enemy camp where he is to be executed. Throughout the passage describing his capture and imprisonment, Shigehira is depicted as weak and passive, no longer the sturdy warrior who earlier had accomplished great feats of masculine strength and bravery on the battlefield.

His new guard, Munemochi, however, was a compassionate man who never treated him severely. He first offered Shigehira a hot bath. In this bath Shigehira thought that he might wash away the dust and grime of the long journey and purify himself to meet the end that could come at any moment. In such sad preoccupation, he was just entering the bath when the door of the bathhouse opened and there appeared a beautiful lady of some twenty years. Her complexion was exquisitely white against her raven locks. She was clad in an unlined silk robe and a blue patterned overwrap, and attended by a maid of fourteen or fifteen, whose hair hung to her waist. The maid was also wearing an unlined white silk robe and a blue patterned overwrap; she carried some combs in a wooden basin. The lady waited upon Shigehira as he bathed. Then, after she had bathed herself and washed her own hair, she took leave of him.

As she was going out, she said to Shigehira: "It was my master Yoritomo, who sent me to serve you here. He sent a woman, because had he sent a man he would be considered lacking in elegance. He also ordered me to ask if there might be anything that

The bathroom of warlord
Toyotomi Hideyoshi at his
Hiunkaku Villa, now located on
the grounds of the Nishi Hongan-
ji temple in Kyoto. The roofed
chamber at left is the steam room;
outside it, water was boiled in
great cauldrons, and shelves were
installed so that Hideyoshi's armor
and weapons could be near at hand
even while he bathed.

he could do for you. Perhaps he thought that a man would have
some difficulty, but that a woman could manage this better."

"Since I am a captive, I must not expect to receive favors,"
replied Shigehira, "but there is one thing I desire—to take the
tonsure and become a monk."

The official history of the new military regime
that Minamoto no Yoritomo established in Kamakura—the
Azuma Kagami, or "Mirror of the East"—records two notable
occasions when charity baths were celebrated by the citizens of
Kamakura. In 1192, Yoritomo ordered one hundred days of
bathing to celebrate the final defeat of the enemy Heike forces
and his successful rebuilding of the Todai-ji temple; each day
one hundred of his retainers bathed. Similarly, in 1239, following the death of Masako, Yoritomo's consort, the military government ordered a period of commemorative baths in her
honor.

The *Hagakure,* a collection of instructions on
proper samurai behavior compiled in 1716 by Yamamoto no
Tametomo, has far more to say about moral rectitude than
about care of the body. Yamamoto offers the example of his own
father as a model of samurai propriety, and the little he says
about bathing is enlightening:

He would get up as early as four o'clock, take a cold bath and
shave the front part of his forehead clean every morning, have
breakfast at daybreak, and go to bed at sundown....

Until fifty or sixty years ago, the samurai would, every
morning, take a tub bath, shave the front part of his head, smoke
his hair with incense, trim his nails and scour them with pumice,
and further polish them with wood-sorrels, being thoroughly
careful not to neglect his personal appearance. Furthermore, he
would dust his weapons and keep them polished and free of rust.

While this particular attention to one's neat appearance
may strike us today as too showy, it does not come from any
romantic idea. Prepared to die in battle each day, samurais,
whether young or old, would keep themselves well-groomed,
because otherwise one's dead body in a battlefield would, betray-
ing his want of preparedness, be surely despised by the enemy as

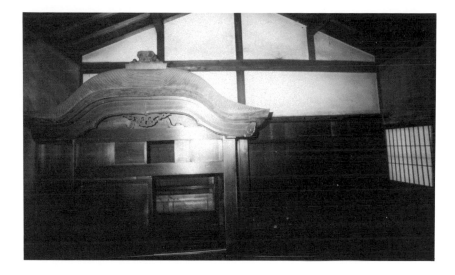

filthy. Though troublesome and time-consuming as the habit
may appear, it is the very thing the samurai is supposed to do;
nothing else in particular demands more haste or time. One can
be free from any danger of shame as long as he, resolutely determined to die at any moment—or thinking himself as one already
dead—strives both in his service and pursuit of military virtue.

In 1600, the warlord Tokugawa Ieyasu suc-
ceeded in consolidating his authority over virtually all the other
military clans and effectively unifying the country. During the
decades immediately preceding and following the establishment
of the Tokugawa shogunate in 1603, Japan was open to European missionaries and merchants. For a time, they were relatively successful in their dual goals of conducting commerce and
propagating Christianity. Most of the European visitors were
Spanish, Portuguese, British, or Dutch, and most shared the
prejudice that their own civilization was far superior to all others and that the Japanese could do no better than to submit to
the enlightening forces of Christian faith and European behavior. Some Europeans, however, were able to see beyond these
prejudices and recognize in Japan a surprising degree of cultural sophistication and social harmony.

From the diaries and other writings of the early
European missionaries and traders emerges a remarkably accurate picture of Japanese society in the sixteenth and seventeenth
centuries. Much of what they saw they considered objectionable,
but in many respects they were highly complimentary. In particular, they were quick to comment on Japanese habits of personal
cleanliness. No doubt, their fascination with the Japanese people's obvious delight in bathing tells as much about the standards of cleanliness of the Europeans themselves as about those
of the Japanese they were observing. Their countrymen in
Europe bathed as seldom as possible and made little effort to
maintain the cleanliness of their bodies or clothes, their homes
or city streets. The habits of the Japanese provided a remarkable
contrast to the general acceptance of filth in contemporary
Europe. Many of the Europeans in Japan were quick to abandon
their own unclean ways and adopt the Japanese ideal of per-

sonal hygiene, and few neglected to comment upon it in their
letters and diaries:

> They wash twice a day and do not worry if their privy parts are
> seen.
> —Jorge Alvares

> Europeans take a bath privately in their homes; in Japan, men,
> women, and bonzes wash in public baths or at night in the
> porches of their houses.
> —Luis Frois, S.J.

> All the homes of the nobles and gentry have bathrooms for
> guests. These places are very clean and are provided with hot and
> cold water because it is a general custom in Japan to wash the
> body at least once or twice a day. These extremely clean bath-
> rooms have matted places where the guests undress for their
> baths. They put their clothes in a place where there are white
> perfumed robes of fine linen hanging up and these they use to
> dry the body after the bath. Clean new loincloths are available,
> and they put them on when they wash and bathe themselves in
> order not to wet their silk ones, which they wear instead of draw-
> ers. There are also perfume-pans which give a sweet smell so that
> the guests can perfume themselves after the bath.
>   Their baths consist primarily of a sudatorium made of pre-
> cious scented wood and other medicinal wood, with a small door
> which they shut behind them when they enter. It is heated by the
> steam of boiling water, the steam entering through a certain part
> and turning into hot dew. In this way the steam so gently softens
> the body that it brings out and loosens all the adhering dirt and
> sweat. On leaving the sudatorium the guests enter a very clean
> room opposite where the floor is made of precious wood and
> slopes slightly so that the water may run away. Here there are
> found clean vessels of hot purified water and others of cold, so
> that everyone can adjust the temperature of the water more or
> less as he pleases. And as they bathe there, all the dirt which came
> to the surface in the sudatorium is washed away leaving the body
> very clean.
>   Pages are in attendance there and look after everything. If a
> guest is embarrassed by the pages of the house, he is attended by
> his own pages; otherwise, those of the house wait on him and
> prepare all that is needed. Some people do not like going into the

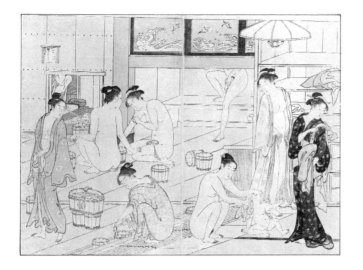

sudatorium and so only bathe themselves with warm water in order to wash away the sweat and refresh themselves, for they say that this way of bathing refreshes the body in very hot weather and warms it in the winter. When many guests go into the sudatorium or bathe together, they observe great courtesies and compliments. This custom of taking a bath is universal throughout all Asia, as is well known from the chronicles. But the Japanese seem to excel everybody else in this matter, not only in the frequency with which they bathe during the day, but even more so in the cleanliness and dignity which they observe in that place, and in their use of most precious and medicinal wood in the construction thereof.

— Joao Rodrigues, S.J.

Their hot springs are of this sort. At the source of a big stream the water is incredibly cold, but a little further downstream it becomes as hot as it was formerly cold. At the place where I stayed, I saw a stream entering the sea at a very rocky part where there was but little sand; in the morning at low tide lukewarm water may be found by digging a few inches into the ground. Both winter and summer, many of the poor men scoop out caves in which they lie and wash themselves for several hours, either at sunrise or at sunset when the tide is low and a stream flows into the sea. Most of the women of that place get into the water at sunrise, or even earlier, and quickly douche their heads three times, even though it may be snowing. They then get dressed, and filling some wooden vessels with water they walk through the streets sprinkling the water with their fingers and reciting some words (which I did not understand) until they reach their houses. They sprinkle this water also in their houses, but I think it must be some sort of devotion as it is not done by everybody.

— Jorge Alvares

Perhaps the most comprehensive picture of Japan during the early Edo period is provided by the German doctor-scientist Engelbert Kaempfer (1651–1716), who was attached to the Dutch trading mission in Nagasaki. With the zeal of an inquiring reporter and with eyes un-shuttered by religious ideology, Kaempfer recorded everything he saw during his investigations of the Nagasaki area and on his two extensive

Netsuke, or toggles, depicting bathers in various poses. *Below:* Woman arranging her hair while holding a bronze mirror. Wood, early nineteenth century, unsigned. *Right:* Woman combing her hair after bathing. Ivory, twentieth century, by Masatoshi. *Far right:* Beautiful woman with homely child before entering the bath. Ivory, twentieth century, by Masatoshi. (*From the collection of Raymond and Frances Bushell*)

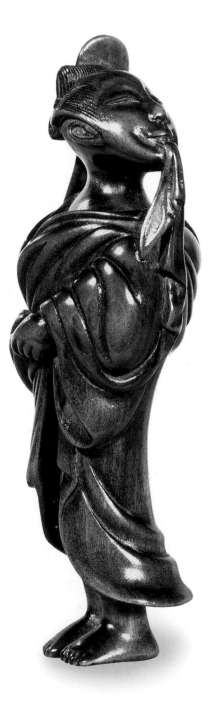

journeys from Nagasaki to Edo in 1691 and 1692. His three-volume *History of Japan* is an extraordinarily detailed and accurate eyewitness report of Japan at a time when few other Europeans were allowed to enter the country (all but the Dutch had been evicted from the country by exclusionist policies of the shogun after 1630). It is clear that Kaempfer's sojourn in Japan was an exceedingly positive experience for him:

> The behaviour of the Japanese, from the meanest countryman up to the greatest Prince or Lord, is such that the whole Empire might be call'd a School of Civility and good manners. They have so much sense and innate curiosity, that if they were not absolutely denied a free and open conversation and correspondence with foreigners, they would receive them with utmost kindness and pleasure.

Kaempfer readily adopted certain habits of Japanese behavior that he found superior to what he was accustomed to at home. He seems to have taken happily to Japanese food and drink, wore Japanese clothes on occasion, and delighted in the Japanese predilection for cleanliness both of the body and of the living environment. He comments repeatedly on the surprising cleanliness of the streets of Nagasaki, Kyoto, and Edo. Of all the contemporary European visitors who wrote about the bathing practices of the Japanese, Kaempfer's accounts are the most detailed:

> The bagnio, or bathing place, is commonly built on the backside of the garden. They build it of cypress wood. It contains either a Froo, as they call it, a hot-house to sweat in, or a Ciffroo, that is, a warm bath, and sometimes both together. It is made warm and got ready every evening, because the Japanese usually bathe, or sweat, after their days journey is over, thinking by this means to refresh themselves and to sweat off their weariness. Besides, as they can undress themselves in an instant, so they are ready at a minute's warning to go into the bagnio. For they need but untie their sash, and all their cloaths falls down at once, leaving them quite naked, excepting a small band, which they wear close to the body about their waste. For the satisfaction of the curious, I will here insert a more particular description of their Froo, or hot-

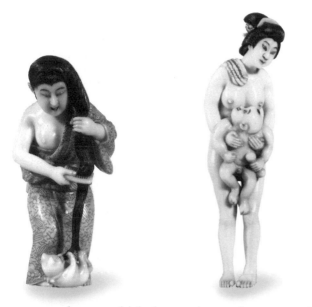

house, which they go into only to sweat. It is an almost cubical trunk or stove, rais'd about three or four foot above the ground, and built close to the wall of the bathing place, on the outside. It is not quite a fathom high, but one fathom and a half long, and of the same breadth. The floor is laid with small plan'd laths or planks, which are some few inches distant from each other, both for the easy passage of the rising vapours, and the convenient out-let of the water people wash themselves withal. You are to go, or rather to creep in, through a small door or shutter. There are two other shutters, one on each side, to let out the superfluous damp. The empty space beneath this stove, down to the ground, is enclos'd with a wall, to prevent the damps from getting out on the sides. Towards the yard is a furnace just beneath the hot-house. The fire-hole is shut up towards the bathing stove, to prevent the smoke's getting in there. Part of the furnace stands out toward the yard, where they put in the necessary water and plants. This part makes all the damp and vapours ascend through the inner tubs, one of warm, the other of cold water, put into these hot-houses, for such as have a mind to wash themselves, either for their diversion, or out of necessity.

In February 1691, Kaempfer accompanied the leaders of the Dutch trading mission at Nagasaki on one of its periodic official visits to the shogun's headquarters in Edo. Such a trip, like the regular mandatory journeys by daimyo and various shogunate officials to and from Edo, was a major undertaking. The distance from Nagasaki is nearly one thousand miles, and the Dutch ambassadors and merchants were accompanied by a large retinue of bailiffs, interpreters, guards, clerks, cooks, porters, and servants. The senior dignitaries rode in palanquins, each carried by two or four porters; the others traveled on horseback or on foot. As they covered no more than thirty or forty miles a day, the trip took nearly a month each way. The slowness of travel afforded the eagerly observant Kaempfer ample opportunity to investigate life along the highways of Japan.

The route from Nagasaki took Kaempfer and his party to some of the famed hot-spring areas of northern Kyushu and, later, to the ancient hot springs of Arima, near

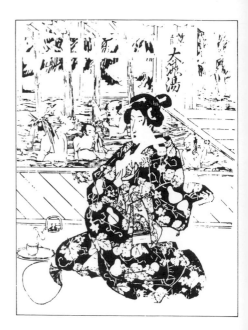

Detail from an anonymous nineteenth-century print depicting the hot-spring resort of Kusatsu. A local beauty sits in the foreground, cooling herself after a bath. Behind her, bathers enjoy the massaging waterfalls that were one of Kusatsu's attractions.

present-day Osaka. With characteristic precision, Kaempfer set down his experiences at these spas. Just north of Nagasaki, at the village of Ureshino, was one of the party's first overnight stops:

> Not far from the village, on the side of a small river which falls down from a neighbouring hill, is a hot bath, famous for its vertues in curing the pox, itch, rheumatism, lameness, and several other chronical and inveterate distempers. This Bath we had leave to see. I found the place rail'd in with Bambous in a very handsom manner. Within the inclosure was a watch-house, and a small booth for the guests to divert themselves. Along one side of the rails was built a long room or gallery, divided into six smaller rooms, or baths, all under one roof. Every bath was a mat long and broad, and had two cocks, one to let in cold, the other hot water, and this in order that everybody might mix it to what degree of heat they can best bear. At the side of this long room was a place for the guests to repose themselves, cover'd with a thatch'd roof. The well was likewise cover'd with a small square thatch'd roof. It is not very deep, but the water bubbles out with great vehemence and noise, and is withal so hot, that none of our retinue had courage enough to dip his fingers into it. I found it had neither smell nor taste and therefore made no scruple to assign its vertues meerly to its heat. The man that shew'd us the place, in order to convince us that there was something extraordinary in this water, pluck'd down a branch of a Camphire-tree (which stood hard by and was about the bigness of a large oak, being the second of an uncommon size we saw since we set out from Nagasaki), dipt it into the hot well, and then gave everyone of us a leaf to chew, which made our mouth and tongue look as if they had been painted with a mix'd colour of green and yellow. Not far from the spring there were two other large baths for the use of poor people. I took notice, that a small brook of cold water, which runs hard by the place, smoak'd in some places, perhaps because of another hot spring in its bed.
>
> There are many more hot wells upon this Island, of the same and some, of still greater vertues. By my repeated and diligent enquiries, I could hear of the following: Jumotto is a hot bath in Arima, which they make use of to cure lameness; another of the same vertue is at Tsuksaki, in the Province Fisen. Another

is at Obamma in the Province Simabara, situate not far from the coasts, and overflow'd in high water. This is but small, shallow, and hath a salt mineral taste, which they look upon in this country as something very remarkable. About three miles from thence, at the foot of the famous mountain Usen, are several hot springs of this kind, within about an hundred paces circumference, all which have a sulphurous smell, and are withal so hot, that no use can be made of them, unless they be mix'd and cool'd by a proportionable quantity of cold water. There was another Pond of warm water at Jamaga in Figo, but it is now dry'd up.

More than anything else, Kaempfer was impressed by the size and scale of activity of the three great Japanese cities of Kyoto (which, echoing his guides, Kaempfer refers to as Miaco or Miyako, "the capital"), Osaka, and Edo. Visiting all three on several occasions between 1690 and 1692, he encountered them at precisely their most intensive moment of urban development. Kyoto, the imperial capital and largest city in Japan since 794, had a population of half a million residents at the time of Kaempfer's visit. Only slightly smaller was Osaka, the center of the rice trade of western Japan and the military headquarters of the warlord Hideyoshi, who had promoted extensive mercantile development there. Fastest growing of the three cities was Edo, which Tokugawa Ieyasu had transformed from a small fishing village to a major urban center when he made it the site for his principal castle and headquarters of his *bakufu* government. Except for the presence of the emperor and imperial court at Kyoto until 1867, Edo was for all practical purposes the capital of Japan after 1600. With the development there of a civil administration that effectively governed the entire country, the population of Edo grew in leaps and bounds: by the time of Kaempfer's first sojourn there in 1691, it numbered half a million; during the eighteenth century it nearly doubled, surpassing London as the largest city in the world, and by the end of the Edo period it had well exceeded a million inhabitants.

Accompanying the rapidly increasing size of Japan's major cities was the exuberant development of a new, com-

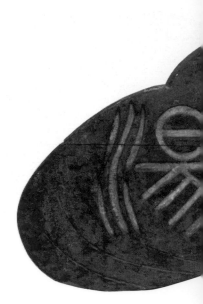

A nineteenth-century *kanban*, or signboard, for a bathhouse in the city of Kanazawa. The inscription, carved in an archaic style, reads *Matsunoyu* (literally, "pine-heated water"), a common name for bathhouses since the pine tree is a symbol of strength, endurance, and longevity. (*Courtesy of Ishikawa Prefectural Museum, Kanazawa*)

74

plex, and highly creative urban culture. Although governed by samurai in a social system inspired by a combination of traditional Japanese military values and archaic Confucian theories of civil administration, the real thrust toward cultural change during the Edo period was borne by merchants, artisans, and other townspeople. The social code of the Tokugawa government, having developed out of centuries of military rule over an agrarian populace, was essentially conservative, and although it successfully resisted change for more than two centuries, in time it proved ill-equipped to address the realities of social change. A rigid class stratification placed the samurai warrior-bureaucrats at the highest level of prestige, followed by farmers and craftsmen, with merchants at the bottom and a still lower subclass that embraced the service personnel, entertainers, and other commoners of the newly burgeoning urban society. The inherent contradiction that the Tokugawa administrators found most vexing in attempting to adhere to this code was that it was the lowest strata that came to provide both the wealth and the creative energy to propel cultural development.

Commercial activity flourished during the long centuries of Tokugawa peace, and the towns and cities provided the perfect setting for the increasingly wealthy merchant class to indulge its taste for sensual gratification. Held in contempt by a Confucian morality that disapproved of avarice and commercialism, and therefore barred from public service and political power, the urban merchants, shopkeepers, and craftsmen (known collectively as *chonin,* literally "townsmen") turned energetically toward the pursuit of luxury, entertainment, fashion, and the cultivation of pleasure as the principal outlet for their wealth.

The urban society witnessed by Kaempfer at the end of the seventeenth century was at the height of its first "golden age." The most colorful symbol of the flourishing urban spirit was the *ukiyo,* or "floating world," the euphemism applied to the licensed pleasure quarters of major cities. From the *ukiyo* flowed the latest fashions cherished by the *chonin,* as

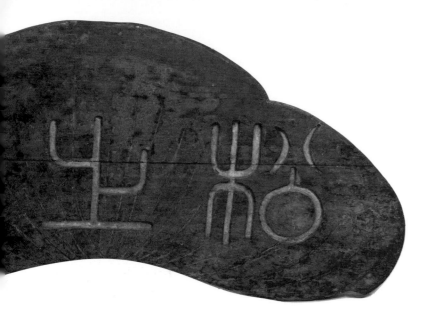

well as the myriad arts and entertainments that animated their lives. Segregated from the austerities of samurai life, the *chonin* embraced the colorful figures of the pleasure districts as their cultural models. It was chiefly the actors and musicians and courtesans who inspired the fashions of the day and who populated the literature and arts that the townspeople found most to their liking. To stem the energetic expression of popular taste, the Tokugawa bureaucrats issued one censorial edict after another and through sumptuary legislation attempted to restrict the craving for luxury among the *chonin* and the flamboyant sensualism of the pleasure districts. But the very repetition of such sumptuary legislation is testimony to its failure. Wealthy merchants required by official decree to wear somber clothing, for example, lined their black kimono with brilliant brocades woven of gold and silver threads; theaters and brothels closed by government edict reopened almost immediately at nearby locations or under different guises; songs or poems or novels banned for their licentiousness reappeared with only a few phrases changed. Despite temporary setbacks caused by official repressiveness and economic depressions, the vitality and creativity of the popular culture continued to flourish and eventually came to prove alluring even to the members of the stern samurai society.

Like the theaters, teahouses, and brothels of the pleasure quarters, the public bathhouses were an important focal point of urban activity. With the dramatic increase in city populations, bathhouses provided an essential social service. Culturally, they offered even more—namely, they helped foster a sense of communal spirit and cohesiveness. As a key meeting place for urban dwellers, the Japanese public bathhouse assumed something of the character of the town green or central plaza of European towns; and as an informal site for the exchange of news, gossip, and ideas, the bathhouses might also be compared to the salons and coffeehouses of eighteenth- and nineteenth-century Europe.

Although the tradition of communal bathing in

Japan began in prehistoric times and was perpetuated in the charity baths of medieval temples and the large pools at hot-spring resorts, the first commercial bathhouse is said to have been erected in 1590 in Osaka. Offering cleanliness to citizens of any social class and for a tiny fee, it was an immediate success. Entrepreneurs in Kyoto and Edo soon afterward opened bathhouses in those cities as well. As urban populations grew with extraordinary speed during the Edo period, the economies of scale offered by the public bathhouses made them an essential feature of urban life. Until relatively recently, only the most wealthy individuals could afford the quantities of fuel needed to provide sufficient steam or hot water to bathe daily at home. At public bathhouses, the cost of fuel, whether it be wood, charcoal, gas, or oil, could be shared by all users. Furthermore, the "democracy of nudity" seems to have held genuine appeal to the Japanese of the Edo period as it does in modern times: with clothing removed, rich man and poor man, samurai and commoner, businessman and beggar are equal in the community of the bathhouse.

To the officials administering the Edo government, bathhouses presented a threat to public safety and general morality, but nonetheless were a necessity that required careful control. The fires that swept through the densely crowded cities were often blamed on sparks from bathhouse furnaces; to contain this danger, regulations required that bathhouses be registered, frequently inspected, and closed on windy days when a stray spark might ignite a holocaust. A more pressing concern of Edo-period bureaucrats, and one that persisted, was the threat to public morality. Although most bathhouses were perfectly wholesome establishments, those near the pleasure quarters were, almost from the moment of their inception, associated with prostitution. Most bathhouses employed young women, known as *yuna,* to assist customers in washing hair, scrubbing backs, washing underclothing, and the like, and in many instances the *yuna* clearly provided other services to male customers as well. In 1600, less than a decade after the first appearance of public bathhouses, a scandalous liaison between a

Edo-period baths as depicted in Japanese films. *Top:* The changing room at a public bath, a step up from the washing area. *Bottom:* A *yuna*, or female bathhouse attendant, bathes a samurai.

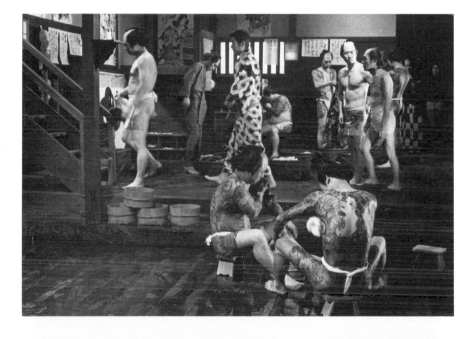

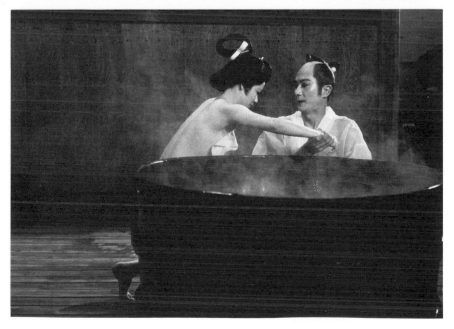

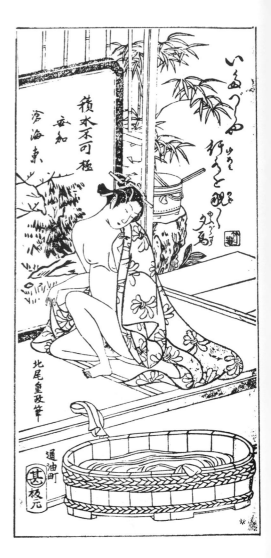

78 samurai official and a *yuna* led to legislation forbidding samurai from frequenting public baths.

The history of bathhouses during the Edo period is a consistent repetition of similar edicts. In 1612, bathhouses in Osaka were distinguished by law from brothels, with both types of establishments requiring different licenses. In 1637, only four years after the appearance of *yuna* was first reported in Edo, bathhouse owners in that city were prohibited from employing more than three of them at one time. A few years later, another edict prohibited customers from staying overnight at bathhouses. In 1648, *yuna* were declared illegal throughout Edo, a proscription that apparently was difficult to enforce since similar edicts were issued at regular intervals thereafter. One technique for evading this kind of legislation was to devise new job descriptions for the female bathhouse attendants: many *yuna,* for example, were renamed *kamiyui-onna* (hairdresser) or *sancha-joro* (tea server).

Alongside the prohibition of female attendants at bathhouses was legislation covering mixed bathing. Attempts to segregate the sexes in bathhouses, initiated toward the end of the eighteenth century, increased in intensity early in the nineteenth, but with little success. Bathhouses, which had been known generally as *yuya* ("hot water establishments") or *sento* ("penny baths"), simply applied for a new license under a different name, such as *yaku-yu* ("medicinal baths"). Although some Western historians believe that the proscription of mixed bathing in Japan was a hasty response by Meiji lawmakers to mollify scandalized Victorians from Europe or America, it is clear from the existence of similar legislation more than a century earlier that such was not the case.

Despite all administrative attempts to regulate their activity, there is no question that public bathhouses were a firmly established feature of Japanese cities throughout the Edo period and into the twentieth century. Their numbers grew constantly until by the mid-1800s there were more than 550 bathhouses in Edo alone. The fees they charged, despite slight fluctuation according to fuel supply, were always so cheap that baths were accessible to virtually the entire populace.

Before the Edo period, the principal form of bathing was the steam bath. Only at hot springs, where natural hot water was plentiful, was it possible to enjoy the special luxury of soaking in hot water. From the beginning of the eighteenth century on, however, bathing by fully immersing the body in hot water became increasingly common in public bathhouses. The 1715 statistics of the Kyoto administrative bureau list fifty-eight establishments of the hot-water type (*yuya*) and thirty-eight offering various types of steam bath (*furo*, the word that in modern times has come to mean bath). In Osaka and Edo as well, hot-water baths rapidly outdistanced steam baths in number. Again, presumably, economies of scale came into play: it was both easier and more economical to heat large quantities of hot water than to maintain sufficiently hot steam in spacious air-tight rooms while customers constantly entered and left. Steam baths were considered more healthful, however, and instead of disappearing altogether they merged with bathhouses of the hot-water type. By the late 1700s, the typical public bathhouse consisted of a large chamber with one or more huge wooden tubs of hot water and a small adjoining steam room. Only a few customers could fit into the small, dark steam room at one time, and they would enter it through the *zakuro-guchi* ("pomegranate door," named for the reddish color of the door's lacquered wood).

By the eighteenth century, bathhouses had already established themselves as neighborhood meeting places. Most were two stories high, with a spacious upstairs room where customers could relax over refreshments and friendly conversation after bathing. So important a feature of urban life were public baths that they became a favorite setting for the lively popular fiction of the eighteenth and nineteenth centuries. Scenes tinged with eroticism in the picaresque novels of Ihara Saikaku (1642–93) and Ejima Kiseki (1667–1736) were often set in bathhouses, where an amorous swain might steal a peek at a

Okumura Toshinobu, *Man on Roof
Looking Through Telescope at Woman
in Bathtub in Garden*, 1730. (*Courtesy
of Tokyo National Museum*)

courtesan he had designs on or a rakish gentleman might entertain his friends with tales of his latest sexual exploits. Just as the
Viennese coffeehouse, the Parisian salon, or the Victorian drawing room might provide the setting for gossip and intellectual
conversation in their respective social milieus, in Edo-period
Japan it was to the bathhouses that townspeople retired for
much of their socializing.

Perhaps the best-known literary work capturing
the atmosphere of the Edo-period bathhouse is the *Ukiyo-buro*
(Bathhouse of the Floating World), written by Shikitei Samba
(1776–1822) in 1810. A brilliant satirist with an ear for collo-
quial speech, Samba took a day in the life of an Edo bathhouse
as a device for caricaturing, one by one, the familiar types of
downtown society. As was common in the satirical fiction of his
day, the preface of *Ukiyo-buro* assumes a tongue-in-cheek mor-
alistic tone, with highflown rhetoric and pseudopious references to the Chinese classics and Buddhist sutras. The full flavor
of Samba's quicksilver style cannot be retained in translation,
but so amusing is this introduction to the colorful world of the
Edo bathhouse that the preface is quoted here in its entirety:

THE LARGER MEANING
OF THE BATH-HOUSE
OF THE FLOATING WORLD

There is, one realizes on careful reflection, no shortcut to moral
learning like the public bath. It is, after all, the way of Nature,
and of Heaven and Earth, that all are naked when they bathe—
the wise and the foolish, the crooked and the straight, the poor
and the rich, the high and the low. The nakedness of infancy
purges them all of sorrow and desire, and renders them selfless,
be they Sakyamuni or Confucius, Gonsuke or Osan. Off with the
wash water come the grime of greed and the passions of the
flesh; a master and his servant are equally naked when they rinse
themselves. As surely as an evening's redfaced drunkard is ashen
and sober in the morning bath, the only thing separating the
new-born baby's first bath from the cleansing of the corpse is life,
fragile as a paper screen.

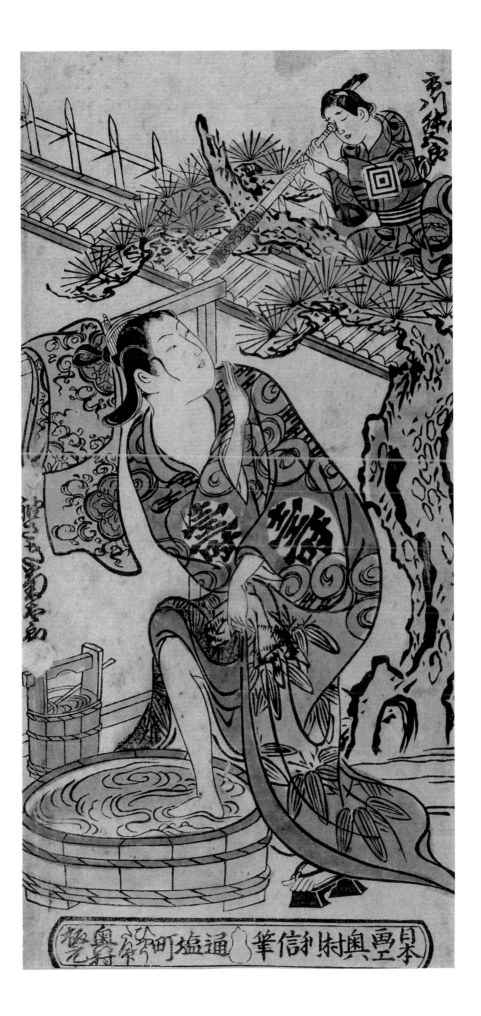

So it is that the old man who loathes Buddha enters the bath
and at once recites a prayer in spite of himself. The rake takes off
his clothes, and for once feeling shame, covers his private parts.
The fierce warrior restrains his anger when someone pours water
over his head, for the place is crowded. And the hotheaded bully,
his arm tattooed with invisible gods and demons, bows when he
goes through the door, and says "excuse me." Are these not signs
of the power of the public bath?

While a man of feeling may have his private thoughts, the
unfeeling bath affords no privacy. Should one, for instance, attempt to fart discreetly in the bath, the water will at once go
"buku-buku," and bubbles will rise to the surface. In his thicket,
Yajiro may do what he likes, but in the larger world of the bath,
will not even he feel shame?

At the bath-house one sees demonstrated every one of the
Five Virtues. Hot water warms the body, removes dirt, cures ills,
and heals fatigue. This is Benevolence. A bather will not touch
another's wash bucket without first asking if it is free; and far
from being selfish with the rinse buckets, customers will hurry to
finish and lend them to others. This is Integrity. Bathers deni-
grate themselves—"I'm just a bumpkin," "Oh, I'm cold-blooded,
I guess"—and politely say to others, "Excuse me," "Good to see
you," and "After you!" Or perhaps they will say, "Come, let's be a
little quieter," or "Go ahead, please take your time." This is
Propriety. The proper use of cleansing powder, pumice stone, or
gourd skin to remove soil, or of cutting stones to trim the hair—
this is Wisdom. Adding cold water when someone finds the bath
too hot, or hot if it is cold, and scrubbing one another's backs—
these things are Trust.

The public bath being this auspicious sort of place, its patrons come to understand, through using the square dipping-
bucket and the round wash-pail, that water does, indeed, con-
form to the shape of the vessel, as the Lotus Sutra teaches. Like
the floor boards of the bath, their hearts are constantly polished,
and the filth of the world cannot long adhere....

The bath-house rules require watchfulness against fire, and
indeed, one must guard against the fires of human passion. The
rules say, "In times of strong wind, the bath may close at any
time"; so it is that when the winds of luxury blow in the heart, a

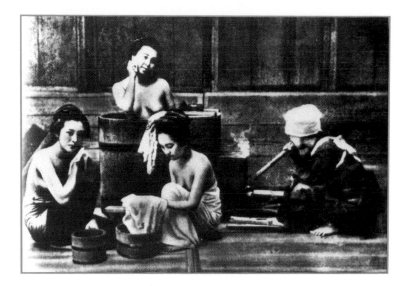

fortune may be lost in a moment. The Five Elements and the Five
Bodily Parts have been placed in our safekeeping by Heaven, and
so we carry with us naturally the "valuables" otherwise prohibited
by the rules. Through wine and lust we are apt to leave behind
consciousness and good sense, cautioned though we are about
"leaving articles behind." And is it not true that we "are strictly
forbidden" to blame on others the ills that we bring upon ourselves? Just as "there shall be no quarrels or arguments," neither
should we pursue worldly fame and gain. "There shall be no rais-
ing of voices," whether in joy, in anger, in sorrow, or in pleasure.
Ignoring these injunctions is as sure to result in loss as going to
the bath-house just before closing time, when one risks wasting
the entry fee should the drain plug be pulled too soon. Chew as
you will on your washcloth, there is no profit in regret!

As a general rule, the human heart is as apt to jump from
good to evil as are the bath-house fleas from Gombei's quilted
coat to Hachibei's silk jacket, or from the country girl's simple
robe to the stolid matron's kimono. The underwear that yester-
day was dropped on the floor may today be placed high on a
shelf: the high and the mighty, the lowly and the poor, are alike
creatures of Heaven's will. But good and evil, rectitude and de-
viance are matters of individual choice. Once one comes to a full
understanding of these truths, they will suffuse one's being like
the warmth of a morning bath.

The body should be put safely away as if in a bath-house
locker, a lock placed upon the spirit, and care taken not to don
mistakenly the wrong one of the six emotions.

"The above rules shall be faithfully observed." So saying,
the chief of the guild of the gods, Buddhas, and Confucius
placed his seal, as large as a "peony cake," on the regulations to
be followed in caring properly for one's single life on earth.

Below: Bathers of the Meiji era. In the upper print, bathers come and go from a semi-Westernized urban bathhouse. In the lower print, six women advertise the pleasures of the hot-spring resort at Kusatsu.

Opposite: Okumura Masanobu, *Courtesan after Bath*, c. 1750. (*Courtesy of Tokyo National Museum*)

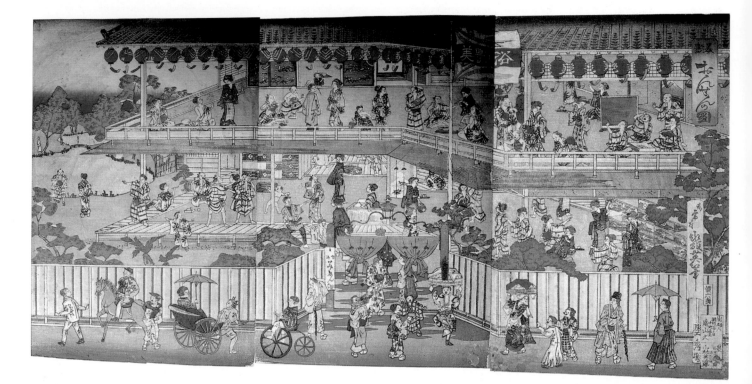

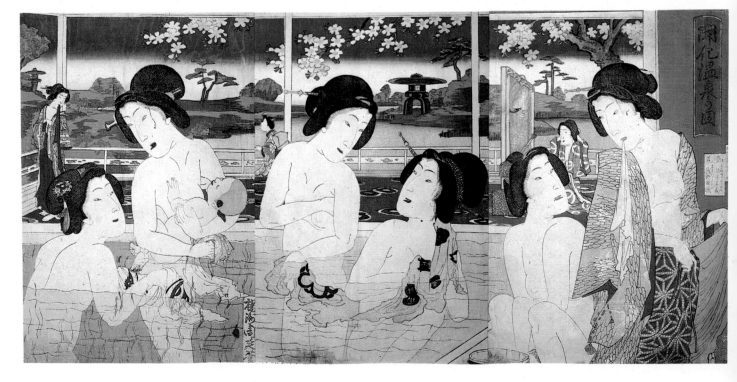

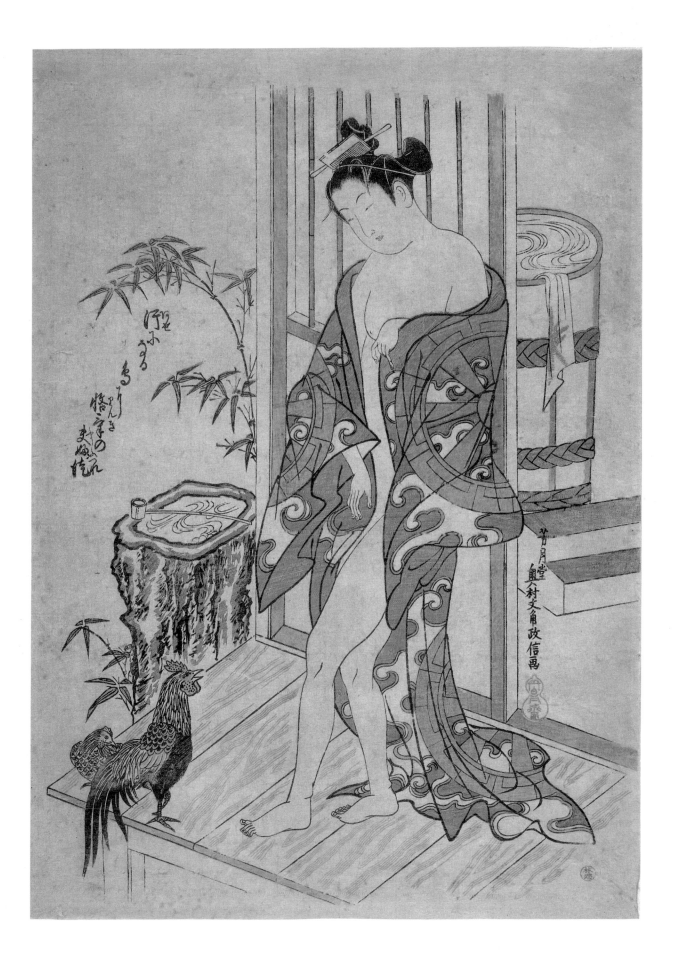

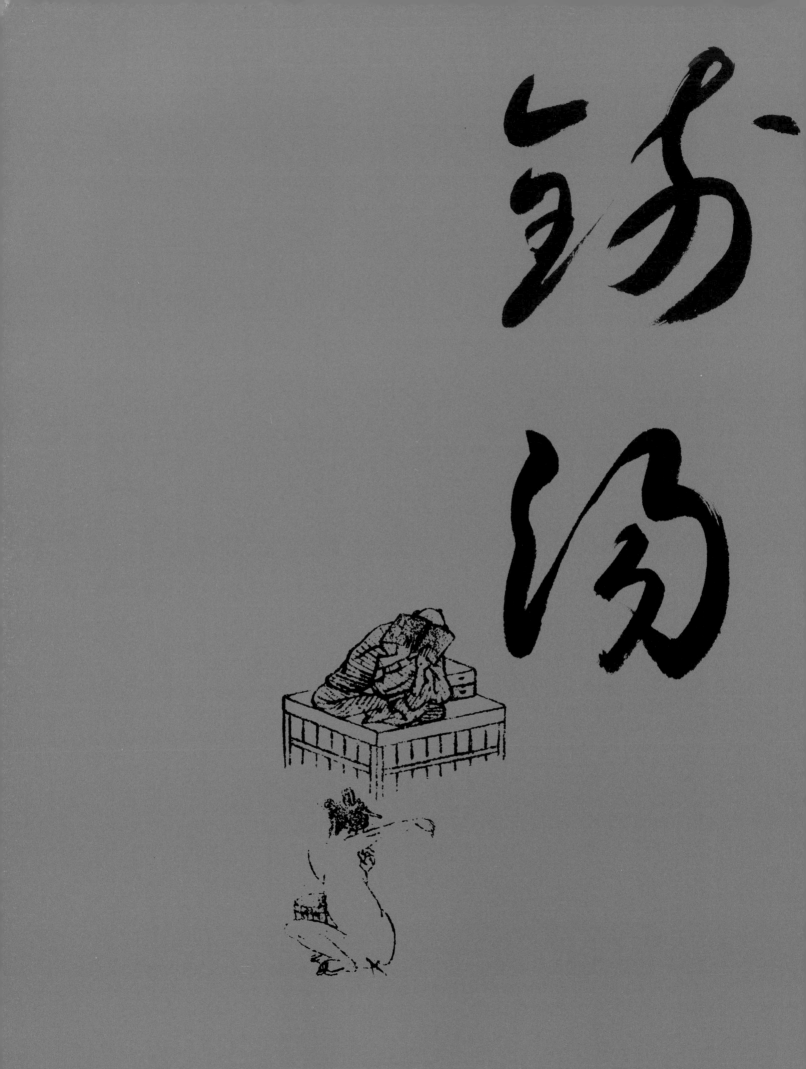

CHAPTER THREE

Public Baths

*S*eldom is heard these days the once-familiar clip-clop of feet in wooden clogs shuffling down the back streets of Japanese cities on their way to the *sento*, or public bath. Disappearing with these footsteps is the rattle of soap in the small basins carried by bathers between home and the local bathhouse. And gone with these sounds is the sight of parents hurrying their children along to the bathhouse or that of returning bathers ambling slowly home, their bodies flushed and steaming, in light clothing even on cold winter nights. Only a few years ago such sights and sounds were commonplace in any residential district of Japan. But today, when more than seventy percent of Japanese homes have private bathrooms, the daily stroll to the *sento* has become little more than a hazy recollection for many modern cityfolk.

Progress moves fast in Japan, but rarely has it whisked so many Japanese along with it as in the past few decades of intense economic development and relatively widespread affluence. Twenty or thirty years ago, only wealthy families enjoyed the luxury of bathing at home. Nowadays, even the most cramped downtown apartment is considered incomplete

Toyohara Kunichika, *Women's Bath*, 1868. (*Courtesy of Maspro Denkoh Art Gallery*)

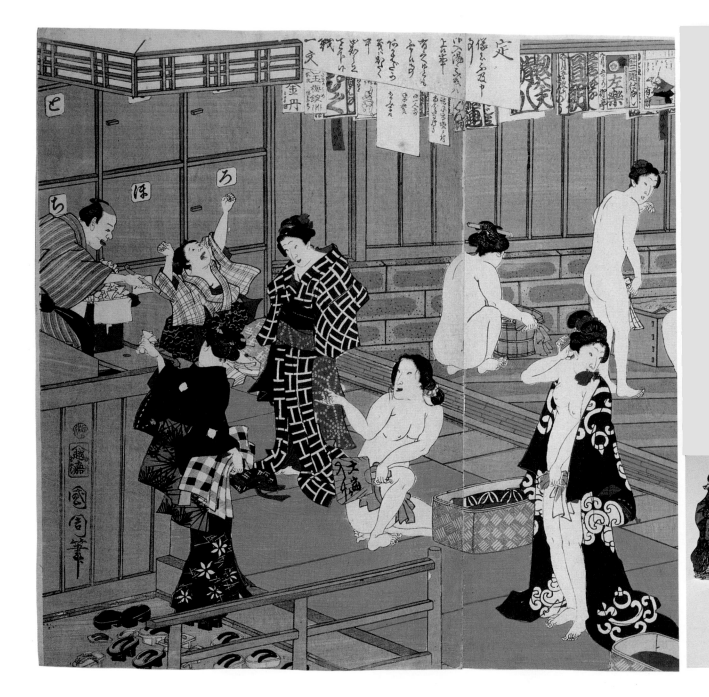

Figures from Katsushika Hokusai's *Manga*, or *Sketchbooks*, populate this re-created scene from an Edo-period bathhouse. (*Courtesy of Ota Museum of Art*)

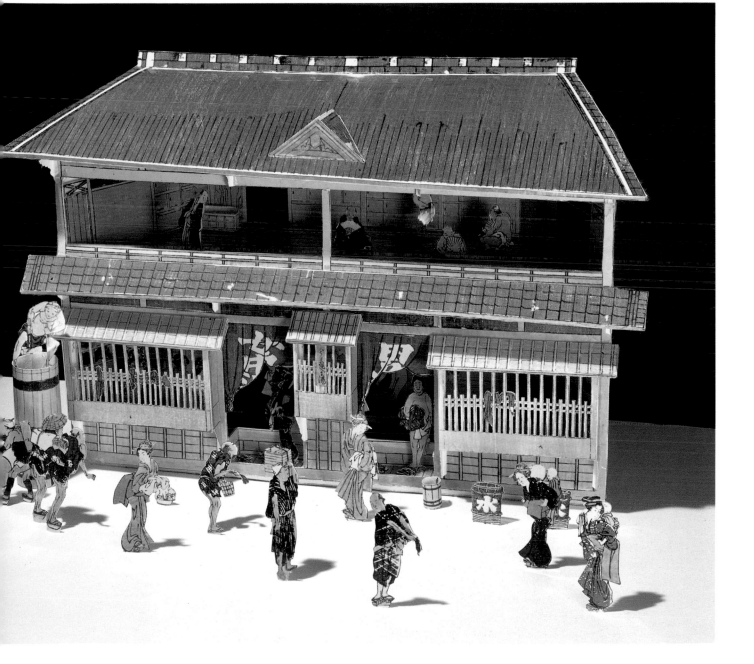

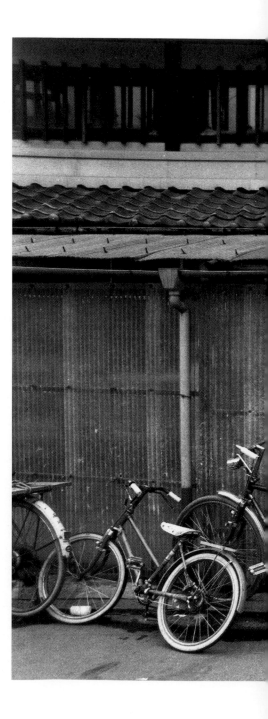

The neighborhood *sento*, or public bath. Shoes and clothing are left in lockers or baskets in a changing room before entering the main bathing area, which is usually separated into men's and women's baths.

without a private bathroom. Clearly, while Japanese families have benefited from having bathing facilities in their own homes, the bathhouse industry has consequently suffered a sharp decline in clientele.

As with so many other features of modern Japanese life, a sense of loss has accompanied the upswing in convenience of daily bathing practices. The feeling goes beyond mere nostalgia. The fact that many Japanese whose homes are equipped with adequate private baths still prefer on occasion to venture out to the local *sento* seems to indicate that bathhouses offer their customers considerably more than simply a bath. Japanese speak of a vague, indefinable loneliness or sense of isolation when they stop going regularly to the *sento*. What they miss can only be the sense of community and involvement in their neighbors' lives that was reinforced by the daily visit to the public bath. In a society where the phrase *hadaka no tsukiai* (literally, "companions in nudity") is used to describe one's closest friends and most informal relationships, their newfound luxury of solitary bathing brings with it a diminished circle of friendships and personal connections.

Japan had nearly 20,000 bathhouses a mere four decades ago. Today that number has shriveled to 12,000, with the decline hastened not only by the loss of customers to private baths but also by the sharply increased costs of fuel and other expenses needed to manage a *sento*. Naturally enough, cities—with their concentrated populations—are the remaining stronghold of the public bath. Tokyo has 2,250 bathhouses today, while many rural communities have none at all. Occasionally a courageous urban bathhouse owner, instead of closing his faltering business and seeking other work, will rebuild or renovate his *sento*, hoping to lure back customers by installing modern devices like whirlpool tubs, saunas, and spray-massage showers. But he is clearly bucking the trend of the times. The great majority of bathhouse owners are more prudently abandoning the hereditary family business for a more lucrative occupation, replacing their *sento* with an apartment house, office building, or other commercially viable structure.

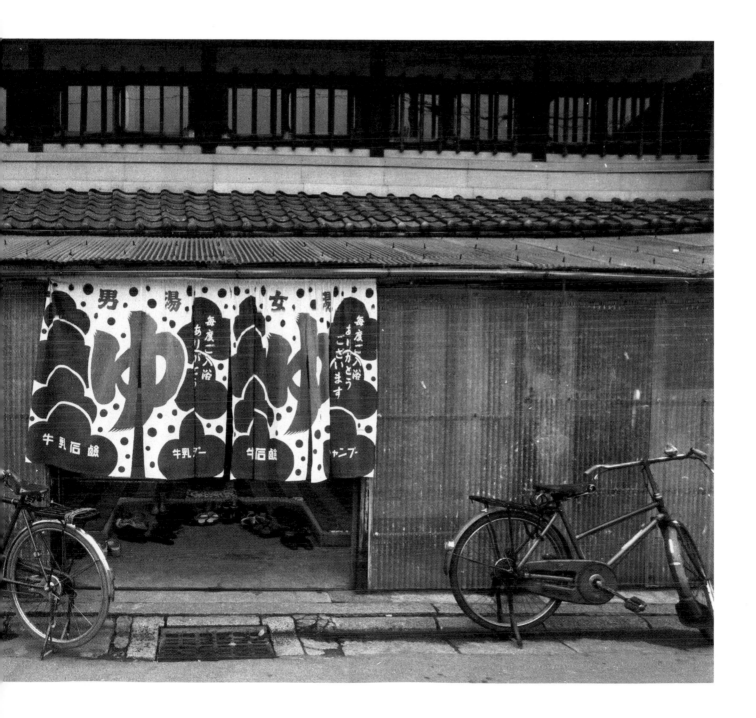

Mermaids lull the bather into a euphoric bliss at the Asakusa Kannon Onsen in downtown Tokyo. Different pools offer water at varying temperatures: from merely hot to scalding.

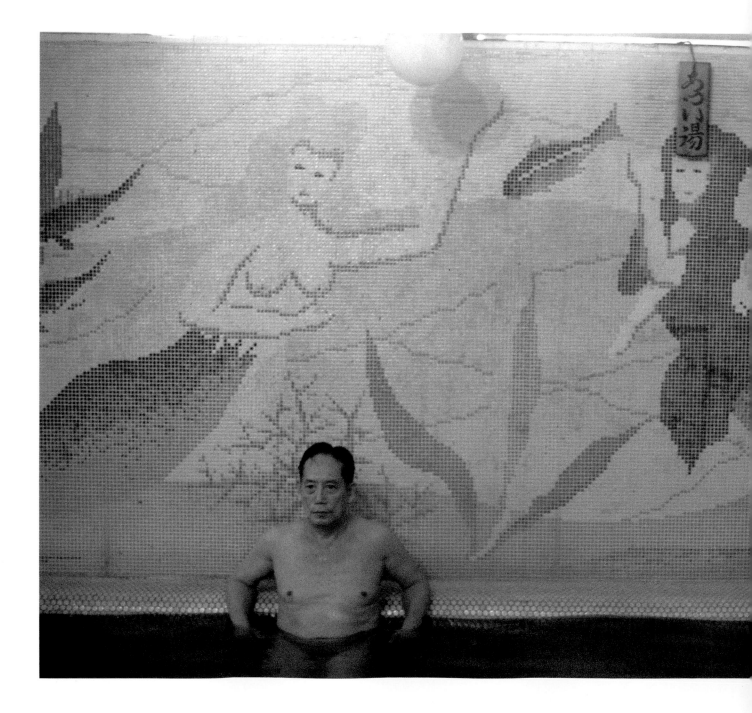

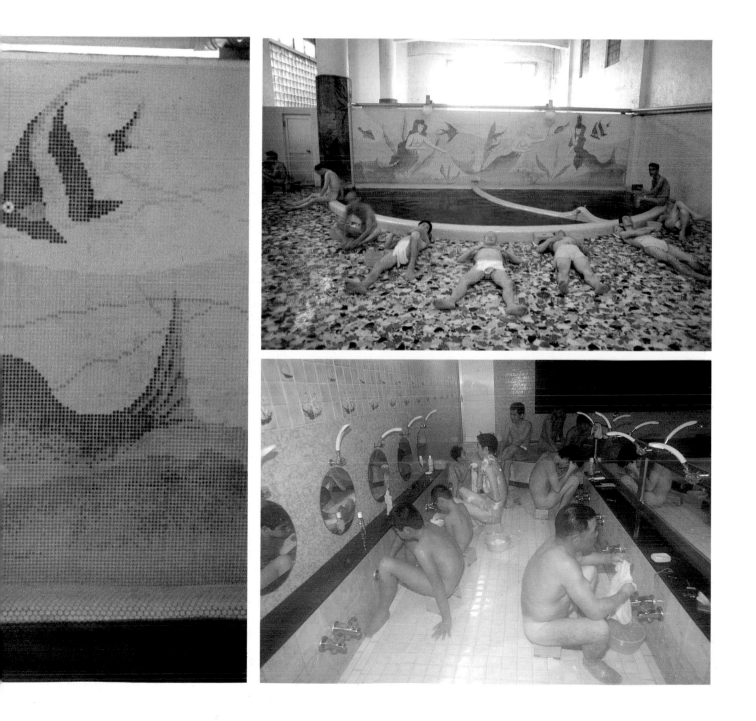

Most bathhouses, responding to such economic strictures, do not open until three or four o'clock in the afternoon, despite occasional pressure from citizens' groups advocating early-morning bathing. According to a popular superstition, the first bather of the morning will enjoy a lucky and prosperous day, a notion that has given rise to citizens' groups with names like *Asa-buro-kai* (Morning Bath Association) who support various social-welfare programs in addition to early bathhouse hours. Nevertheless, such groups are limited in size and influence and they alone cannot guarantee the survival of the bathhouse.

Despite their steady decline in recent decades, the function and form of public bathhouses have remained basically the same over the past few centuries. The provision of bathing facilities—their ostensible function—has been almost secondary to their role as neighborhood centers where friends meet to exchange news and gossip and where the myriad relationships that bind a community are strengthened every day. In the past, bathhouses also offered their patrons a variety of leisure activities that had little to do with bathing. Most had a large second-story room where customers would retire after the bath to eat and drink, play games, or simply engage in relaxed conversation. Several modern-day Tokyo bathhouses have preserved the clubhouse atmosphere of these second-story chambers by adding a small stage where patrons—particularly elderly men and women with time on their hands—can watch occasional variety shows or entertain themselves with their own songs and dances. But the majority of city bathhouses, single-story structures for the most part, provide more modest entertainment in the form of massage chairs, cold drinks, electronic game machines, and magazines.

In form, modern bathhouses have maintained many of the fundamental features of their Edo-period antecedents. Their interior space is divided into a small anteroom, where patrons leave their shoes and umbrellas; a large dressing room, presided over by the proprietor or his wife, who collects the entry fee (approximately \$1.00 in Tokyo today) and sells

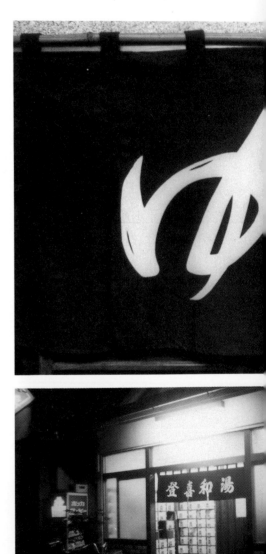

Scenes at the *sento*. Bathers arrive on foot or on bicycle and shed their shoes at the entrance. Just inside the front entrance, seated on a dais overlooking both the men's bath and the women's, the bathhouse proprietor collects admission fees and sells soap, shampoo, and other sundry necessities.

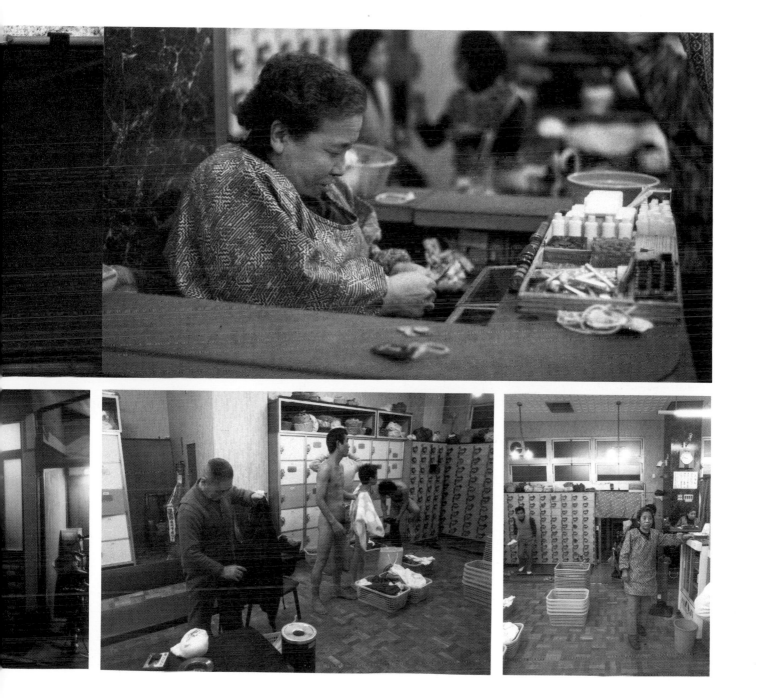

More scenes from the *sento*. At rare
moments it is possible to find solitude at the public bath, although
noisy splashing and chatter usually
enliven the atmosphere.

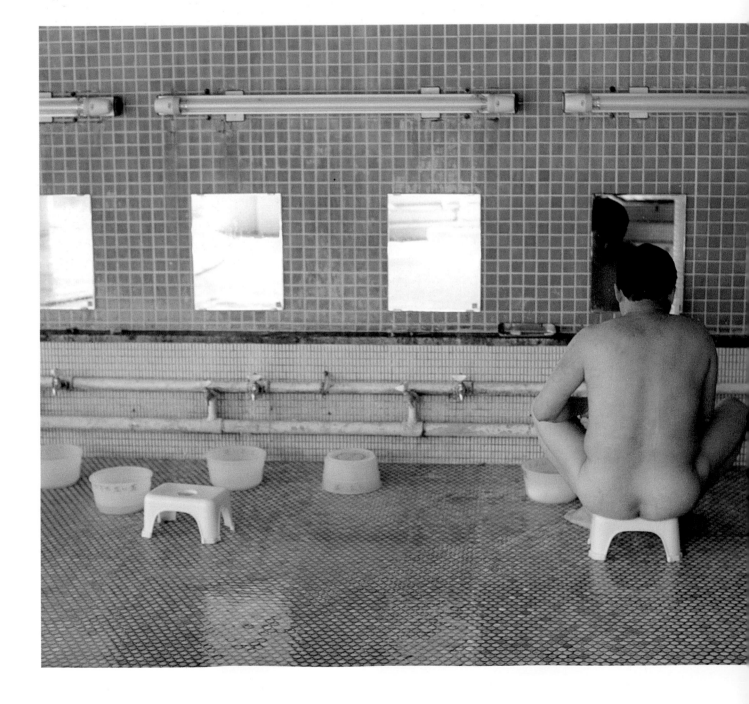

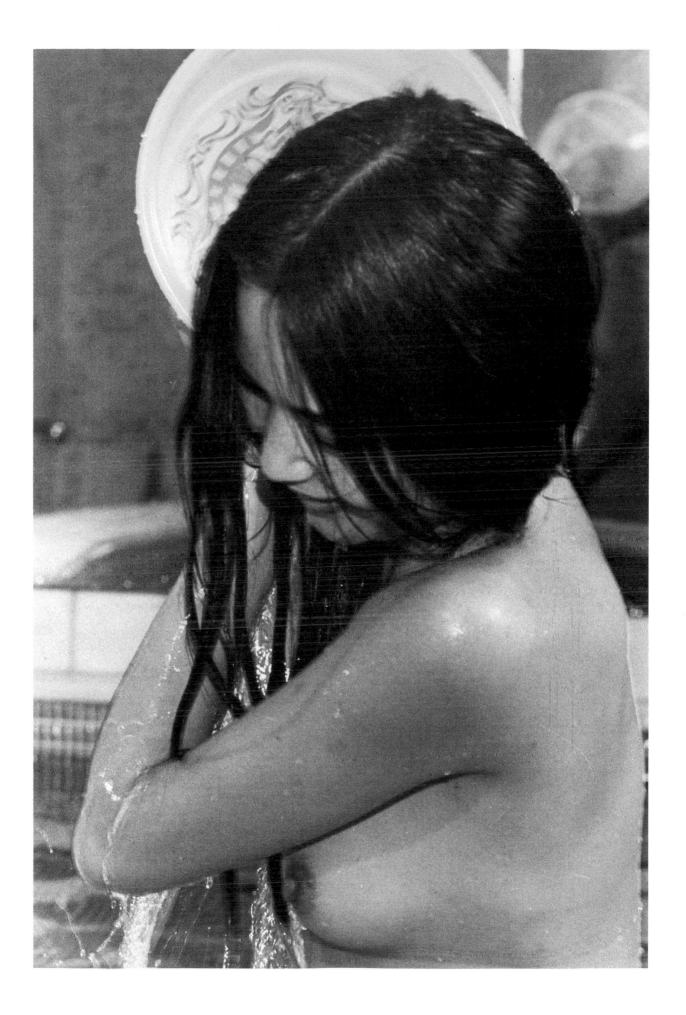

Tokyo Onsen, one of the largest bathhouses in downtown Tokyo, is crowded around the clock. The bather in the foreground "wears" the elaborate full-body tattoo favored since the Edo period by firemen, laborers, and gangsters.

soap, shampoo, razors, and other necessities; and a large bathing area, with faucets and showers lining the walls and two or more deep pools of varying temperature for soaking in. By law, temperatures must be at least 42° C (107.6° F), a considerable drop from those prevalent in the seventeenth and eighteenth centuries, when citizens of Edo (present-day Tokyo) took great pride in braving scalding waters. Ever since the influx of Western medical knowledge in the late 1800s, warning of the dangers of exceedingly hot water on those suffering from high blood pressure, temperatures in Japanese bathhouse tubs have fallen steadily.

Two notable changes distinguish modern *sento* from earlier models: nearly all bathhouses today are divided down the middle into a men's section and a women's section (mixed bathing has virtually disappeared from public baths); and the steam baths prevalent in the early Edo period have given way to hot-water baths, a change that was nearly universal by the middle of the nineteenth century. While early bathing rooms were divided into two sections—a general washing area and a dark inner steam room—today the partition has been eliminated, leaving a single large tiled area where washing and soaking takes place under bright illumination.

The long struggle against mixed bathing (and against the licentious activities that were its almost inevitable side-effect) was finally won by government authorities around the end of the nineteenth century. Inordinately sensitive to the reactions of European and American visitors who objected to displays of public nudity, Meiji officials strengthened legislation banning mixed bathing. Through the stringent regulation of bathhouses, they were finally able to enforce these laws to a degree that had eluded their Edo predecessors. Western observers were persuaded to consider Japanese increasingly civilized and respectable as the practice of mixed bathing faded away. Although they display no particular prudishness, Japanese men and women bathe together only at the occasional hot-spring resort that is today, for better or for worse, the exception to the rule of segregated baths.

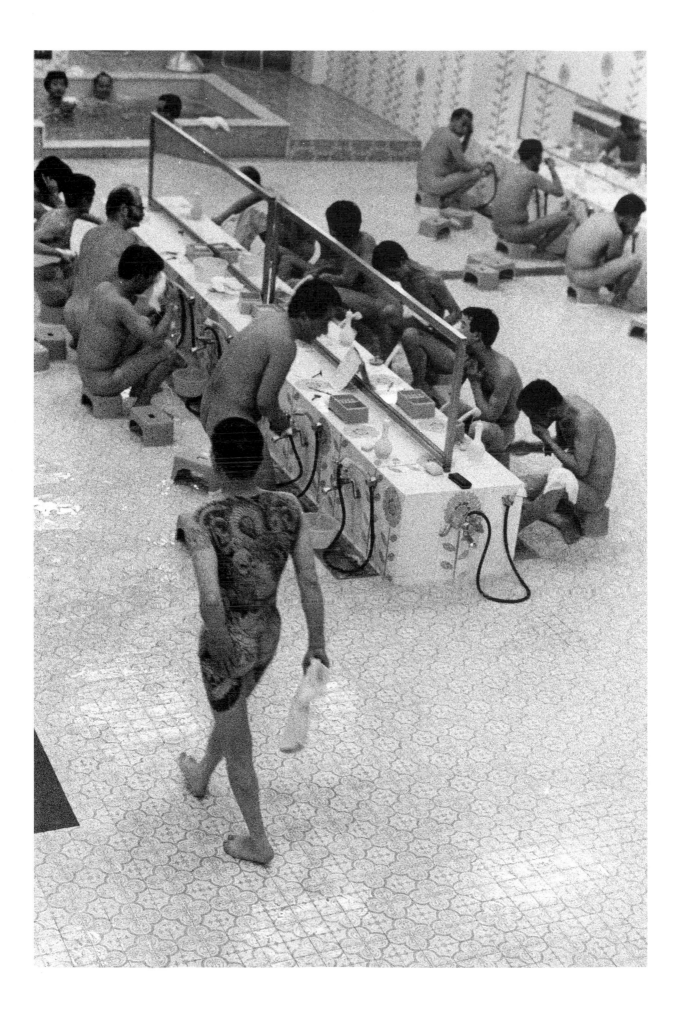

At old-fashioned baths, where hot water is not available from faucets on the wall, bathers scoop the water they need directly from the soaking pool. Since all washing is done outside, the pool remains clean.

One feature common to Edo-period baths that has disappeared altogether is the presence of bathing attendants. Following the repeated proscription of the services of female attendants, male attendants, known as *sansuke,* became a standard feature of premodern bathhouses. They assisted bathers by scrubbing their backs, giving massages, tending the fires that heated the water, and performing other necessary but altogether innocent services. For some reason, most *sansuke* seem to have come from the coastal district of central Japan known as Etchu (modern-day Toyama, Ishikawa, and Fukui prefectures). In time, some of them, who were initially the lowliest employees of the bathhouses, usurped the positions of their masters. Today, many of the families operating Tokyo bathhouses trace their origins to bath attendants who emigrated from Etchu in the sixteenth or seventeenth century.

Another aspect of early bathhouses that has almost entirely disappeared is their access to natural surroundings. Edo bathhouses, even those in crowded urban districts, were usually built adjoining a carefully tended garden. Patrons could enjoy a view of the garden from a broad veranda, or they might stroll through it scantily dressed while they cooled off from the steam or the hot water. Today, no city bathhouse enjoys the luxury of space given over to a garden. Instead, nature has entered directly into the bathhouse in the form of the colorful landscape mural that seems to be an obligatory feature of modern bathhouse decoration. Favorite scenes, rendered in bright pigments or colorful tile mosaics, include: Mt. Fuji; a sunrise over the famed "wedded rocks" of Futami-ga-ura; and the pine-clad islands of Matsushima (one of the "three loveliest landscapes" of traditional popular lore). Some bathhouse owners of less traditional taste have decorated their walls with fanciful underwater scenes of tropical fish and mermaids or with such famous international vistas as the Blue Grotto of Capri, the Swiss Alps, or the beaches of Waikiki. Such mural landscapes may be combined with more lifelike symbols of nature—potted palms and ferns that flourish in the warm, humid atmosphere of the bath. But always there is some token connection with

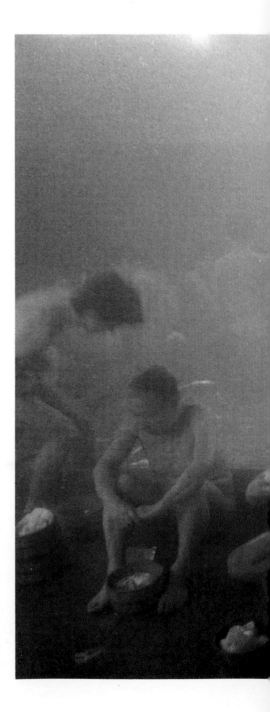

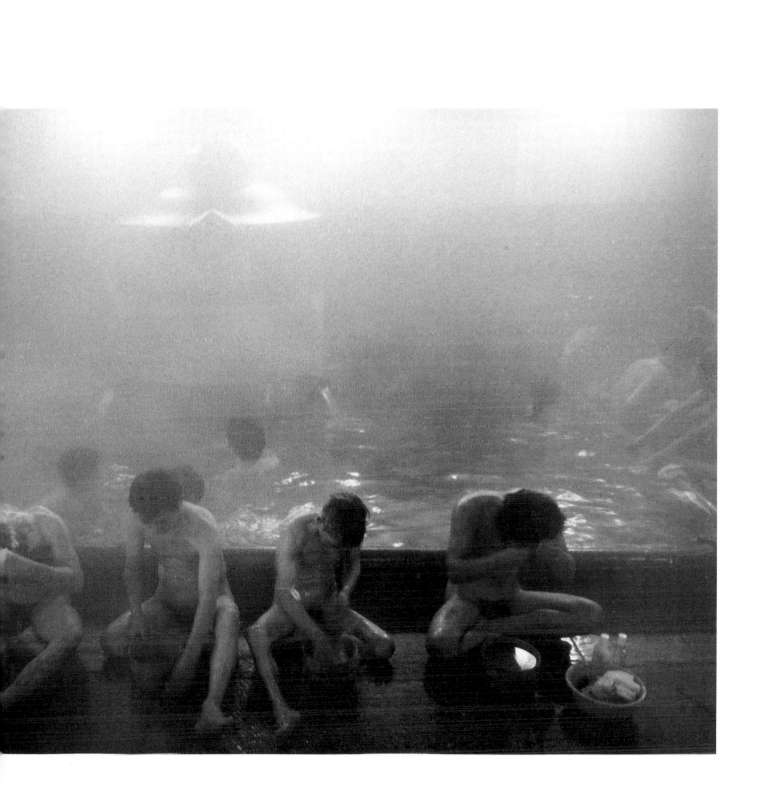

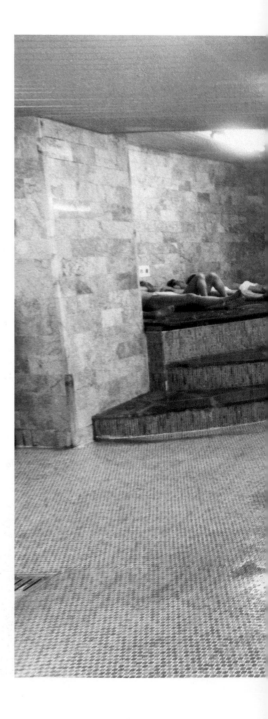

Modern bathhouses provide abundant hot water, individual showers, steam rooms and saunas, and mirrors everywhere. This spacious facility is located within Tokyo Station, offering travelers an opportunity to clean and refresh themselves after a long train journey.

nature, a conscious or unconscious reminder of the bather's identity as one of the myriad inhabitants of the natural universe and of his primordial habits of bathing in hot outdoor springs.

The public bath has given rise to two ubiquitous items of everyday use in Japan—the *yukata,* a lightweight summer kimono, and the *furoshiki,* a square cloth for wrapping and carrying objects. The former originated in the *yukata-bira*—literally, "hot-water robe"—which was a simple garment of ancient times worn in the bath in compliance with Buddhist scriptures forbidding skin contact with others. While the emperor bathed in a robe of silk, the average citizen wore a *yukata-bira* of white linen. Washing the body while garbed in a full-length kimono was no easy task, so sometime around the thirteenth century bathing garments were reduced to a *yu-fundoshi* ("hot-water loincloth") for men—a strip of cloth wrapped around the lower torso—and a *yu-maki* for women—what amounted to a wraparound skirt. The *yukata* continued to be worn as an after-bath garment for helping absorb remaining moisture and perspiration stimulated by the steaming waters. By the time nude bathing made its appearance in the early 1700s, the bathing loincloth and skirt had become underwear for men and women, respectively. Gradually, as the *yukata* evolved into homewear, the Japanese started decorating the somber white fabric with summery patterns and motifs. On sweltering summer nights the *yukata* was donned for a stroll in search of cooler environs. Today, the *yukata* is a summer kimono, most commonly of blue-and-white cotton, that is worn during summer festivals, around town at hot-spring resorts, as loungewear at Japanese inns, and, as in times past, for strolls of a midsummer's night.

Public baths are also credited with popularizing the *furoshiki,* a square cloth that, in skillful hands, can be used to wrap and carry virtually anything. The first popular use of *furoshiki* was at public bathhouses in the early 1600s. Not only were personal articles transported to the bathhouse in *furoshiki,* but *furoshiki* were also spread on the floor (thus their name—literally, "bath spread") so the bather could dry his feet and lounge

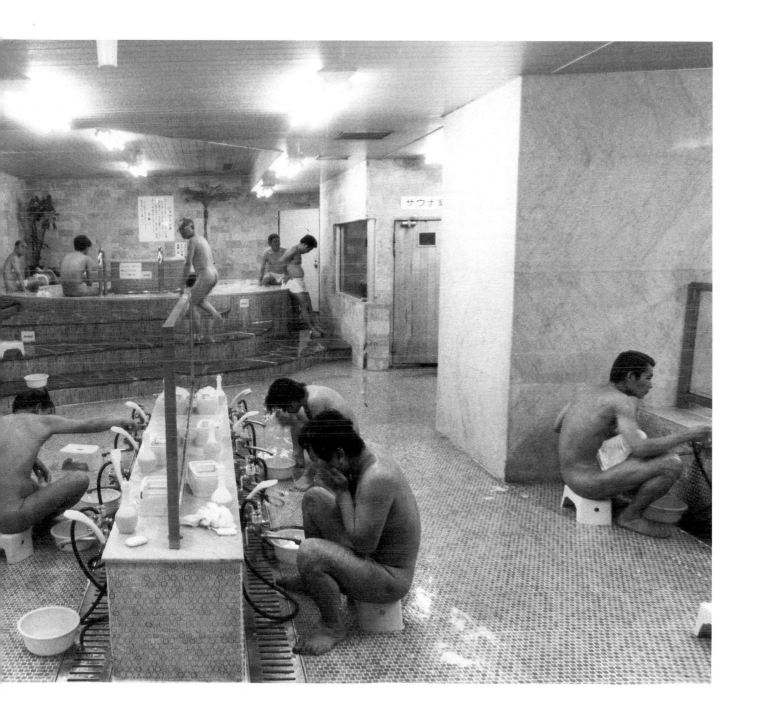

Japanese ablutions are not casual. Before indulging in a long soak in deep hot water, bathers carefully scrub and rinse every inch of their bodies.

Overleaf: Even urban bathhouses, far from the forested glades of mountain hot springs, have a natural setting of sorts: they are usually decorated with potted plants, trees and mosaic murals of famous landscapes (often far more realistic than the flower design seen here). The sign over this bath at *Tokyo Onsen* explains the functioning and health benefits of this new type of bath introduced from the United States—the Jacuzzi.

on top of it as he cooled down and dried off after his bath. To avoid confusion in the changing room, *furoshiki* were dyed different colors or family crests were added—decorations that are still common today in the cloth's modern reincarnation as a substitute for a shopping bag or handbag.

The atmosphere prevailing in modern Japanese bathhouses is not much different from that so vividly described by Shikitei Samba, Ihara Saikaku, and other popular Edo writers of picaresque fiction: raucous, high-spirited, and joyful. The sensual pleasures of warmth and cleanliness seem to bring out the best in people: the Japanese respond with happy chatter and contented sighs. The smooth floors and walls of tile magnify the din of spirited conversation punctuated by splashes and the high-pitched laughter of children. The sounds of the bathhouse change with the shifting cycle of the daily clock, beginning relatively quietly in midafternoon, when the doors open to the first customers—generally, elderly retired folk eager for the company of other senior citizens. Later in the afternoon, the decibel level rises as the bathhouse fills up with children home from school and young mothers bathing babies before going home to begin preparing the evening meal. The noise reaches its highest pitch during the evening hours when older children come for their baths, along with fathers and young single men and women, many of whom may have thrown back a drink or two on their way to the bathhouse. By ten-thirty or eleven at night, quiet begins to fall over the bathhouse again as weary shopkeepers or late-returning office workers enjoy a relaxing soak before drifting home to bed. The last sounds of the day are the gurgle of the drains, the splashing of water, and the swishing of soapy brushes as the proprietors and staff scrub the floors and tubs and rinse away the aftermath of one long day and prepare the bathhouse for the next.

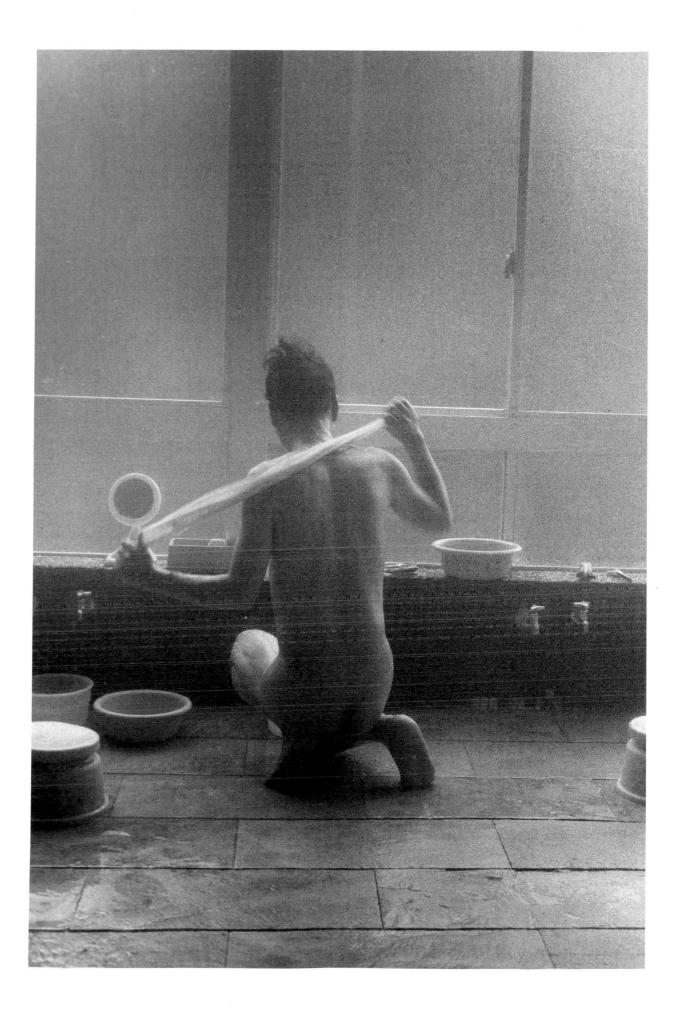

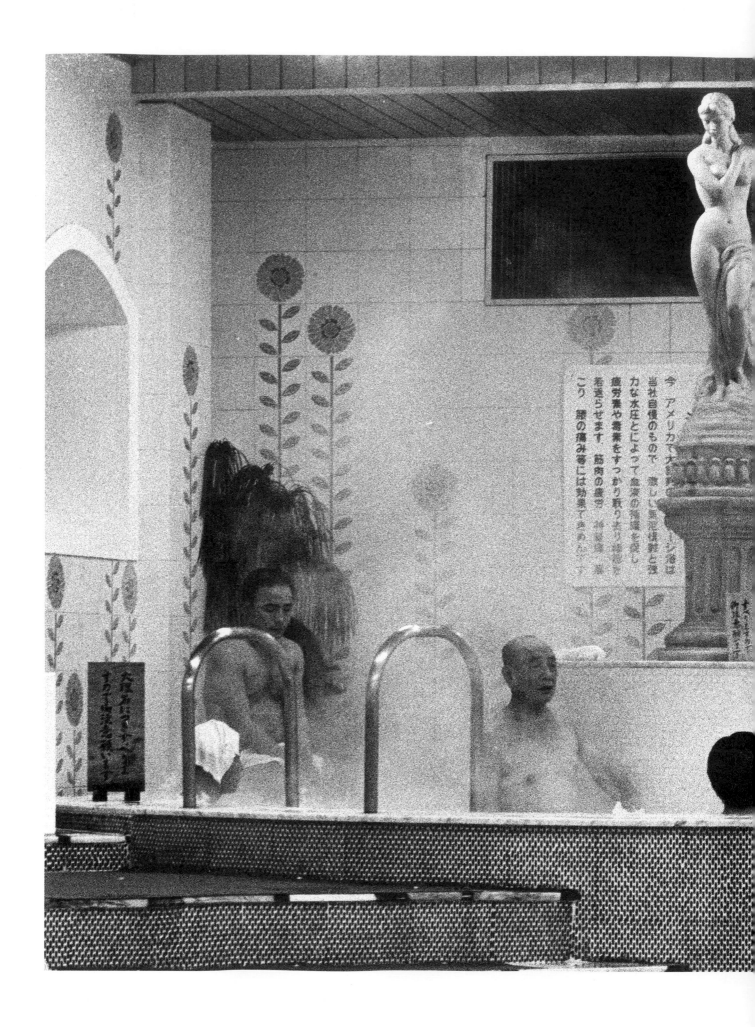

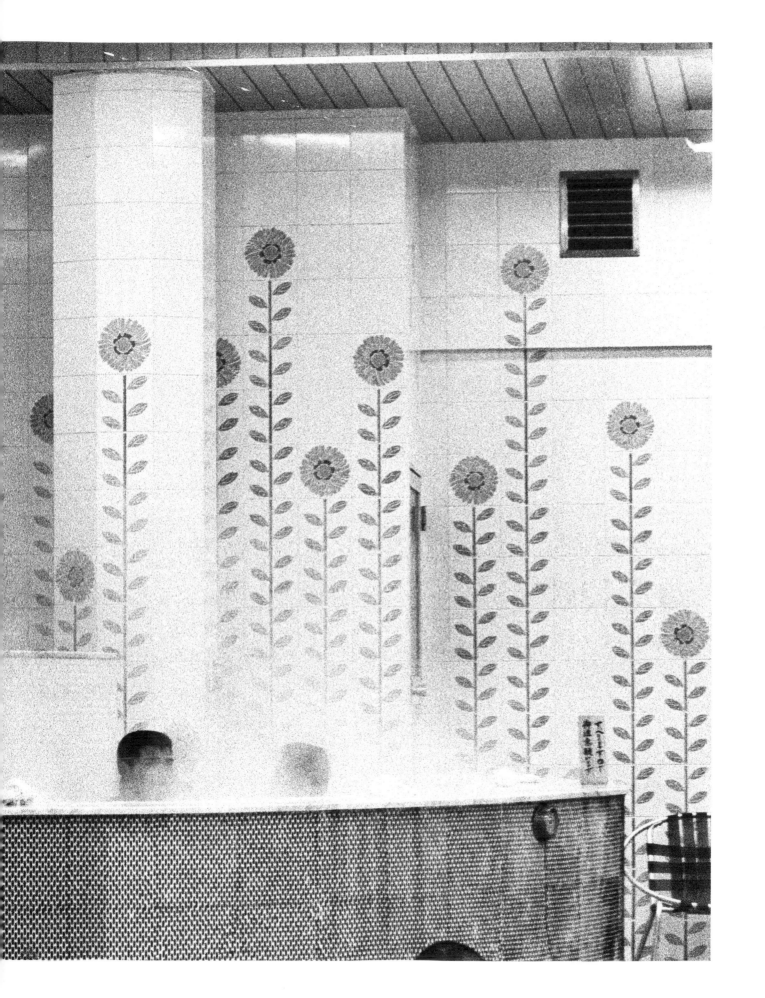

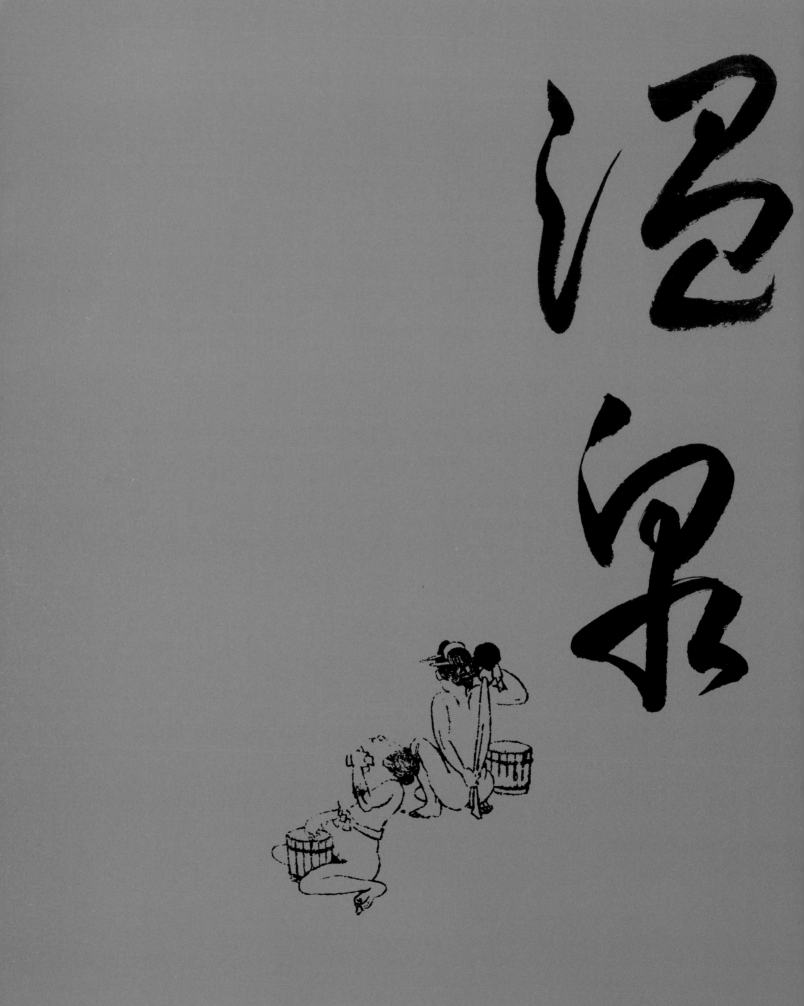

Onsen: The Hot-Spring Bath

Bathed in such comfort
In the balmy spring of Yamanaka
I can do without plucking
Life-preserving chrysanthemums.

—Matsuo Basho
The Narrow Road to the Deep North

*O*nsen, the natural mineral hot springs with which Japan is so richly endowed, represent bathing at its simplest and its most glorious. The varieties of *onsen* are virtually infinite, ranging from isolated spring-fed pools in wooded thickets deep in the mountains—no people, no hotels, no entertainment, no sign of human hand save a worn path trod by hunters, woodcutters, campers, and other bathers—to crowded cities given over entirely to the pleasures of hot-spring bathing—hordes of boisterous vacationers, hundreds of hotels with huge bathing chambers, neon-lit casinos, and dark alleys offering entertainment of every sort and price. And everything in between.

Since time immemorial, *onsen* have been valued by the Japanese for their salutary effects on both body and spirit. When early hunters came across injured deer or other animals nursing their wounds in hot-spring pools, they took instruction from nature and followed course. Calling these springs *kami no yu*, or "divine bath," they believed the waters had supernatural powers to cure illness. For this reason, the origins of many hot springs are attributed in legend and folklore to kindly saints of healing or holy men of exceptional virtue.

Many of the hot springs are alleged to have been discovered or created by the monk Gyoki (668–749), best known for supervising the construction of the great bronze statue of the Buddha in Nara at the behest of Emperor Shomu in the middle of the eighth century. He was considered qualified for that massive undertaking by the sanctity acquired in his lifelong career of good deeds. Chief among these were his legendary feats of bringing forth healing hot water from rocks as he traveled on foot all over Japan. Kobo Daishi (774–835), an equally saintly figure in Japanese history and founder of the Shingon sect of Japanese Buddhism, was also believed to have created many hot springs in his wanderings as a mendicant monk. Frequently, according to popular belief, he would encounter diseased or freezing beggars along the road and, feeling compassion for their plight, would strike his staff upon a rock from which a warm spring would miraculously issue forth.

Doctors ministering both to the physical ailments of court nobility in Kyoto and to the mysterious depressions, or "demonic possessions," that afflicted their spirits would prescribe rehabilitation at a hot spring far from the city. No doubt the fresh food of the countryside and the tranquility of the natural environment proved as beneficial as the healing properties of the mineral waters. To anyone able to afford the leisure and the travel, visits to hot springs such as Arima, Tamatsukuri, and Iyo, which had been popular since long before the court was established at Kyoto in 794, were eagerly sought-after retreats from everyday life. Those less affluent found equal relaxation and pleasure at hot springs closer to home.

Japanese warriors, like the knights of Europe and the Indians of North America, were aware of the healing properties of mineral baths, and history offers many examples of their soaking in hot springs to restore their energies. Perhaps the earliest such reference is to the barbarian-quelling campaigns waged against the aboriginal tribes of the northeastern frontiers by the protohistoric general Sakanoue Tamuramaro.

The following array of antique postcards testifies to the popularity of hot-spring resorts. Some resorts offer such exotic attractions as sand baths, waterfall massages, or outdoor pools where wild monkeys or bears may join human bathers. But the principal appeal of all *onsen* is simply the spiritual and physical revitalization derived from relaxing in nature's bountiful hot water.

THE VIEWS OF SHIRAHAMA, YUSAKI.

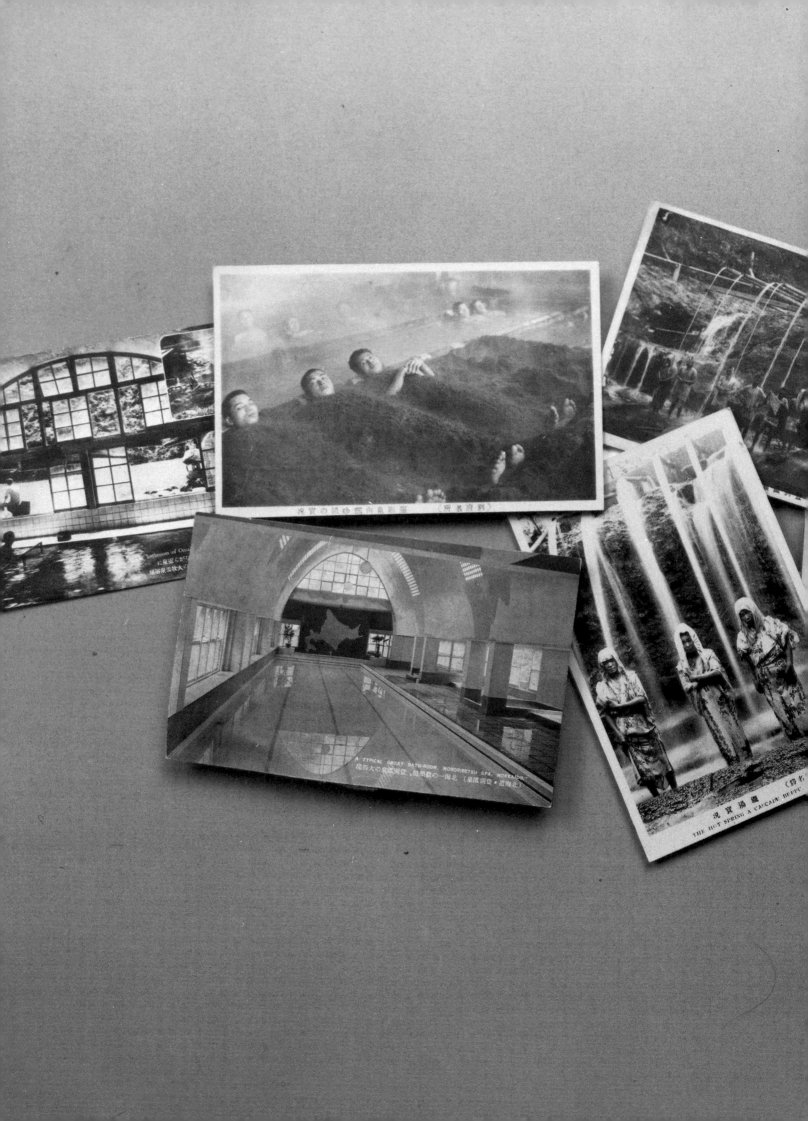

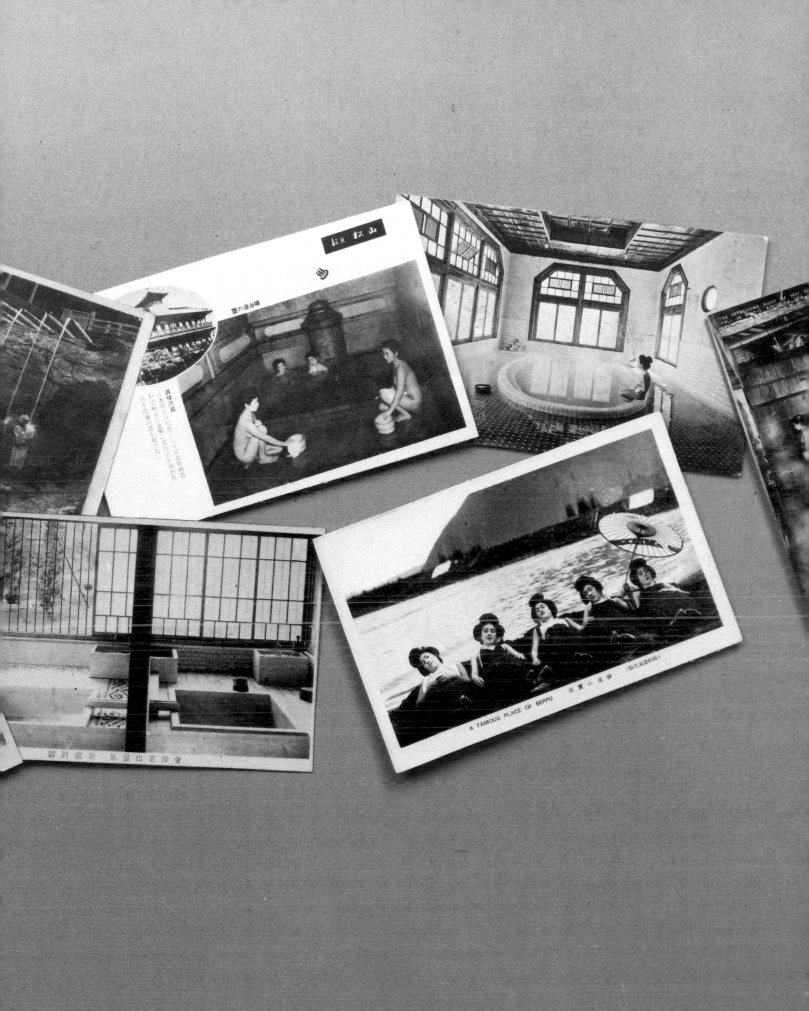

A FAMOUS PLACE OF BEPPU

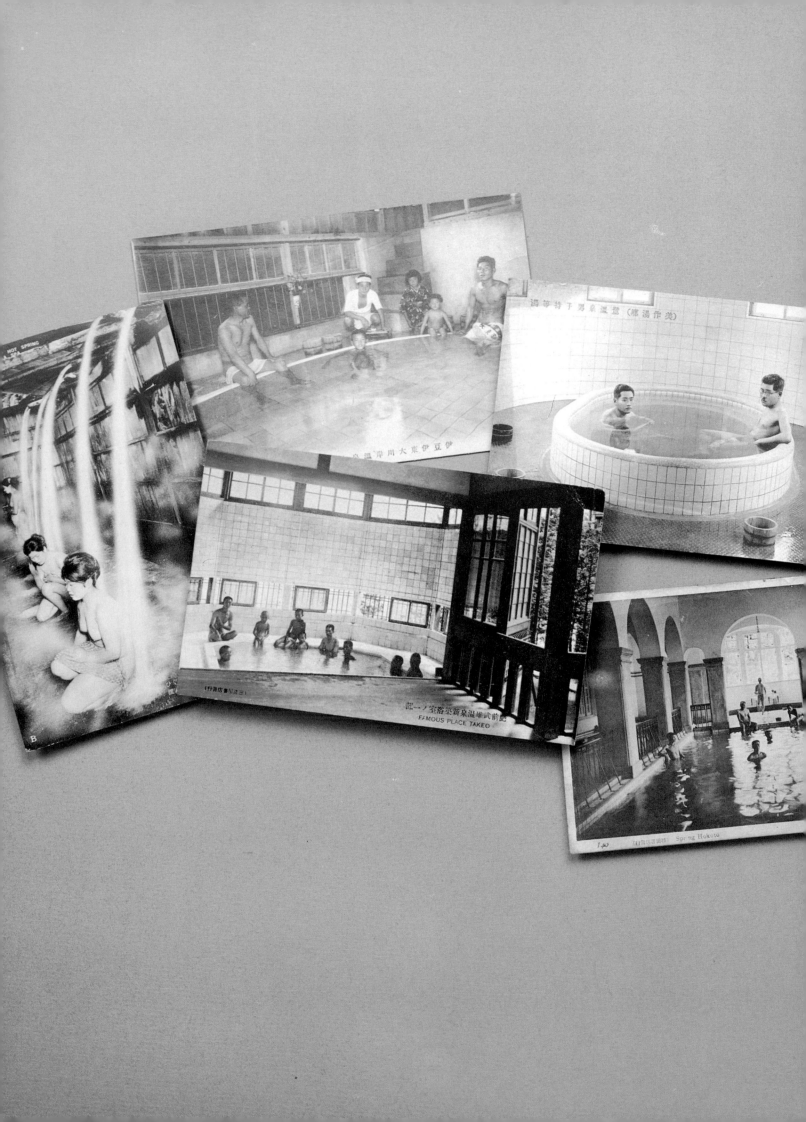

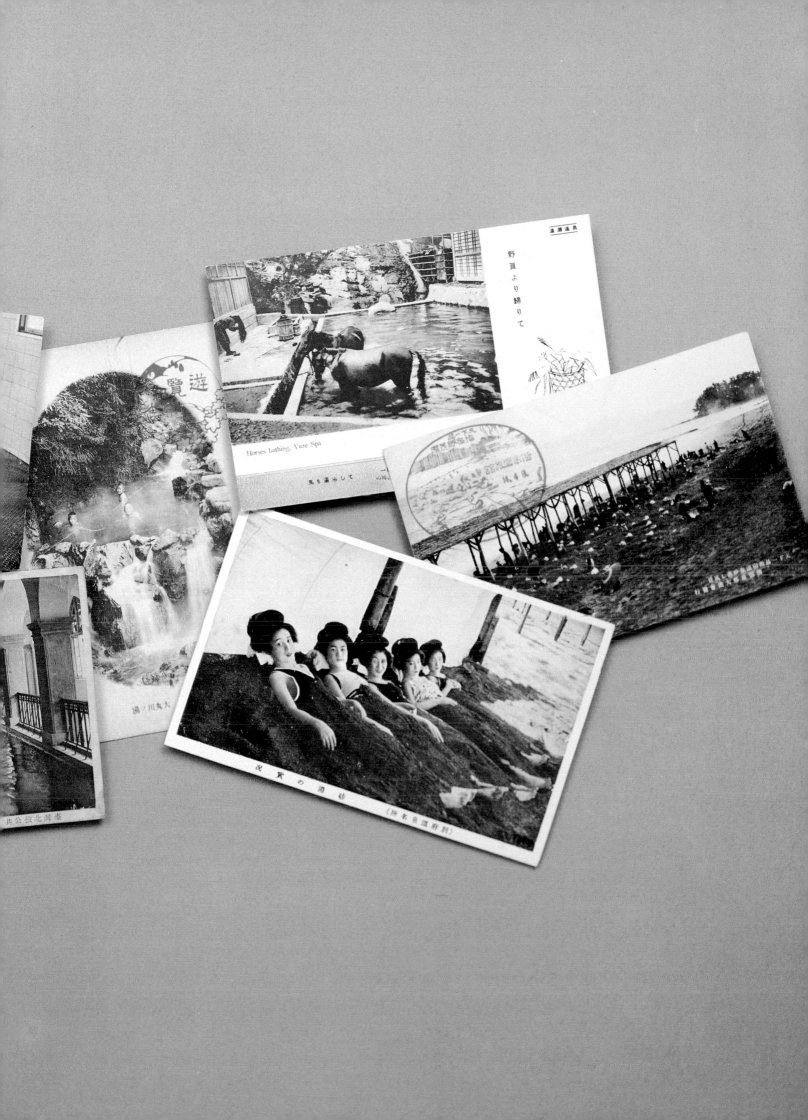

野瀬温泉

野頁より歸りて

遊覽

大丸川ノ渦

Horses Lathing, Yuze Spa

して湯やし馬

共公投北潟壺

砂浴の實況
(別府温泉名所)

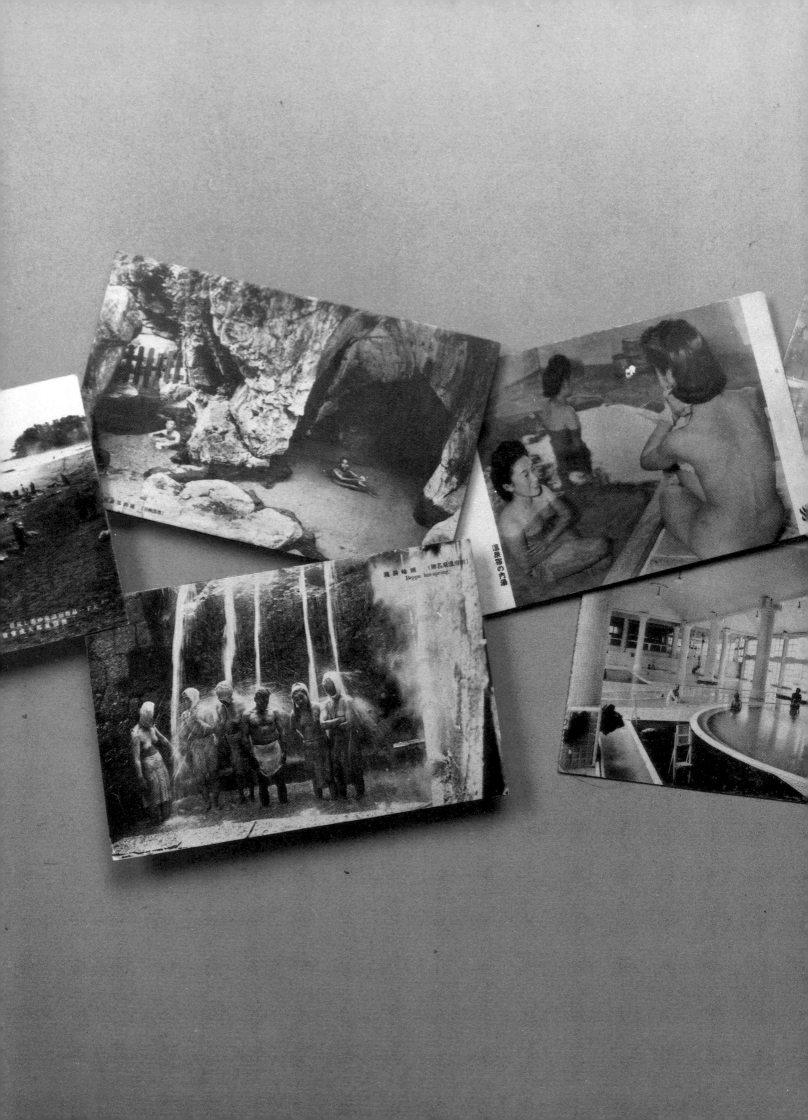

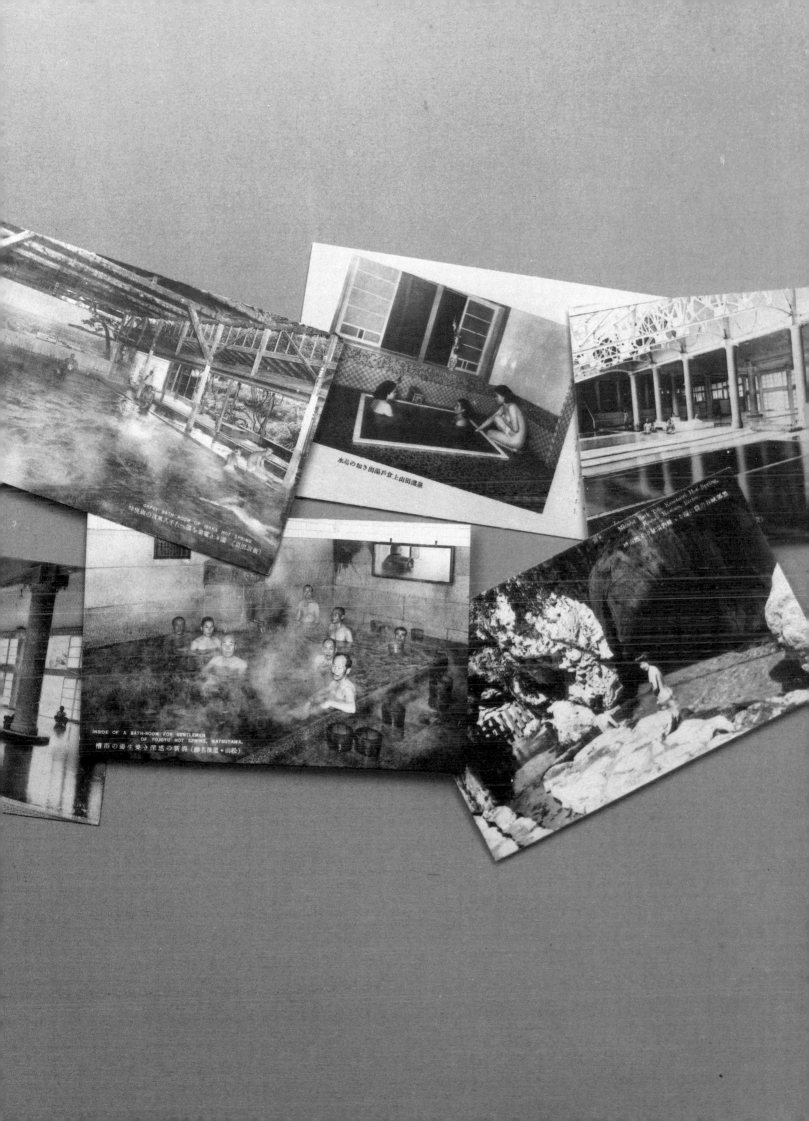

Many *onsen* visitors first encounter the resort town at the square in front of the train station, where buses and taxis wait to convey them to their hotels and where a large map indicates all the nearby scenic spots and sites of interest. Typical of many hot-spring resorts is the cluster of hotels on both banks of a small river running through town. At night, the town's back alleys turn into a colorful maze of neon-lit bars and other enticements for visitors bent on merrymaking.

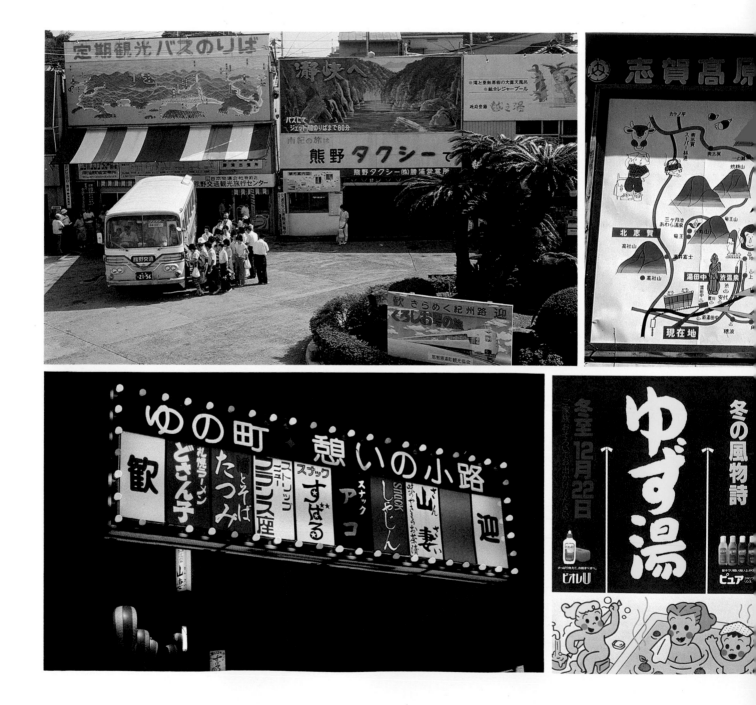

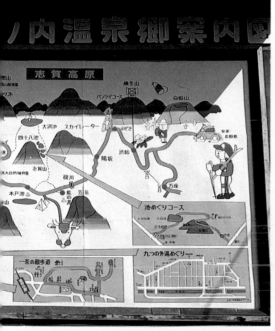

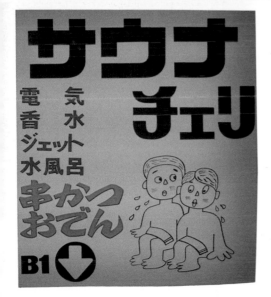

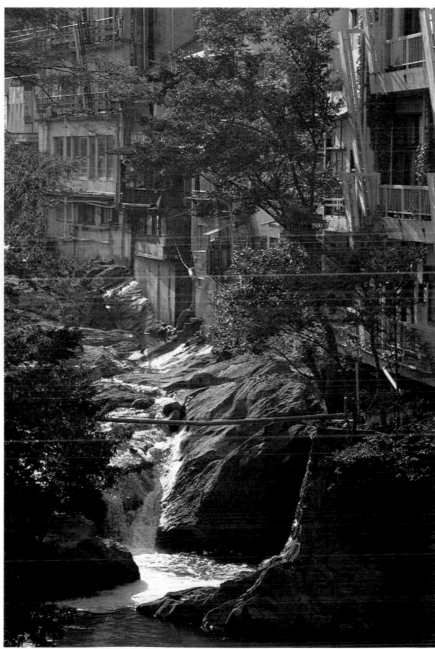

120

After a victorious battle in what is present-day Iwate Prefecture, Tamuramaro is said to have rested his armies at the hot spring of Shidotaira. Centuries later, after history began to be recorded, the mighty Minamoto no Yoshiie (1041–1108) is believed to have temporarily halted his famous campaign against the traitorous Abe clan in order to permit his weary soldiers to regain their strength at Tsunagi springs near the modern city of Morioka. Indeed, the spa takes its name from the spot where Yoshiie tied his horse (*tsunagu* means "to tie or fasten") when he alighted to enter the bath.

The great sixteenth-century warlord Takeda Shingen (1521–73) is known to have carefully exploited the hot springs around his castles and encampments near Mt. Fuji. Calling them "secret springs" *(kakushi-yu),* he developed hospital-like facilities at several such sites. Shingen would send fallen soldiers to heal their wounds at these springs, which were well concealed from the enemy, and he allowed exhausted battalions to rest there briefly before summoning them back to the battlefield. Shingen himself went into seclusion at Yamura *onsen* twice in 1548 to recover from injuries suffered in battle. In 1561, he built a lodge for wounded soldiers at Kawaura *onsen* on the banks of the Fuefuki River; the one hot-spring hotel at Kawaura today is still managed by the descendants of the lieutenant whom Shingen charged with operating that early hospital four centuries ago. The legend surrounding the original discovery of the hot spring at Kawaura is also representative: falling sick on a tour around Mt. Fuji in 1194, the courtier Hatakeyama Shigetada had a feverish dream in which Yakushi Nyorai, the Buddhist healing saint, appeared and urged him to bathe in the river nearby; he did, and quickly recovered. Another of Takeda Shingen's favorite retreats, the hot spring at Shimobe, traces its origins back into prehistory: a hunting party during the reign of the mythical Emperor Keiko (A.D. 71–130) is said to have wounded a deer, which bolted away through the forest; tracking it, they finally found the animal nursing its injuries in a hot spring that, centuries later, is still in use. In more recent times, the U.S. military forces used a number of Japan's well-

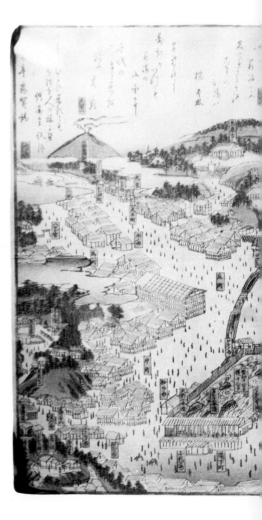

and distant Mt. Fuji on the left. *Right:* Dated 1817, this print lists the fifty-one leading *onsen* in Japan, divided like the lineup for a sumo tournament into Eastern and Western camps. Kusatsu, one of eastern Japan's top-ranked resorts, is listed first at the upper right corner.

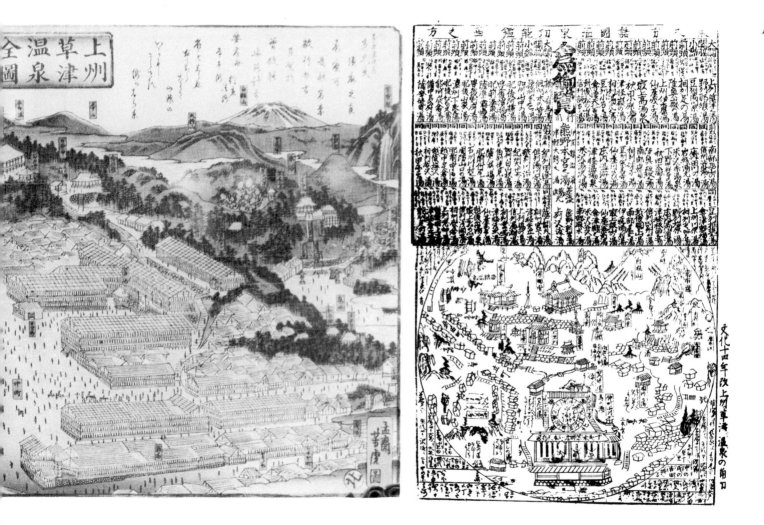

Scenes, old and new, of Kusatsu.
From left: A print by Utagawa
Kuniyasu depicts denizens of the
resort against a backdrop of its
famous waterfalls and spas.
Kusatsu's springs, among the hottest in Japan, must be stirred (and
thus cooled) before bathers can
enter them. This has given rise to a
colorful "water churning" dance.
In the town's central plaza (*far
right*), Kusatsu's scalding springs
send steam billowing into the
night sky.

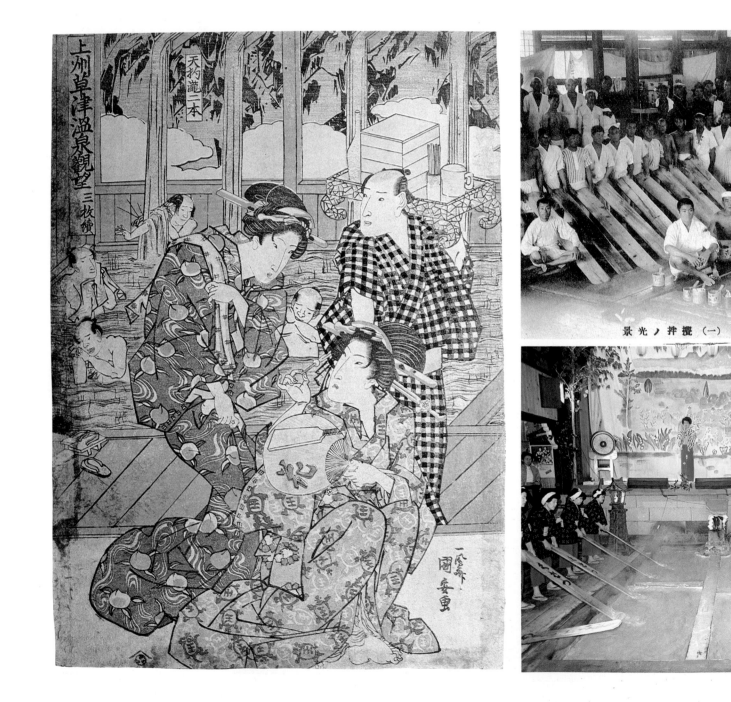

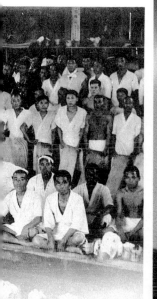

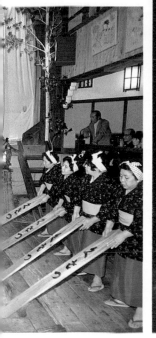

上州草津温泉

123

124

The unpainted wood that encloses Hoshi's hot-spring pools and provides flooring and wall paneling lend the bathhouse a warm, rustic air. The damp, steamy wood emits a pleasant natural fragrance, and the only sounds piercing the clouds of steam are the constant trickle of water and an occasional happy laugh or sigh of a contented bather.

known hot-spring resorts (Hakone, Unzen, and Beppu among them) to provide R & R (rest and recuperation) for American servicemen during the Korean War.

In premodern days, before leisure had become the privilege of all classes and before such expensive amusements as international travel and golf had come into the reach of most citizens, hot springs were the only universal luxury enjoyed by Japanese of all walks of life. The hot water from natural springs cost nothing and could be found almost everywhere. Even the poorest peasant could lay down his hoe at the end of a hard day's work, strip off his ragged clothing, and bask like a king in the fresh hot water bubbling forth in a nearby riverbed or even in the middle of his field. Lowly foot soldiers could set aside their weapons after combat and soothe their aching muscles in a hot spring near the battlefield, and itinerant beggars, mendicant monks, and weary travelers on foot could do the same. Aristocrats, powerful warlords, and wealthy merchants might travel in comfort to distant hot-spring resorts, lured by attractions unavailable to them at home, but neither wealth nor leisure was a requirement for enjoying the salutary blessings of a long soak in refreshing hot water.

Few places in volcanic Japan do not have a hot spring within easy reach. Hot-spring guidebooks are published in great quantities by the Japanese tourist industry; the very number of these books bears testimony to the extraordinary popularity of *onsen* resorts. They list more than two thousand such resorts, the term stretched to include even settlements with only a single hostelry to accommodate bathers. But remove the inn or hotel, and the number of hot springs in Japan soars beyond measure. Many are no more than an enclosure of rocks along a river or a leafy natural pool in a forest, either where hot water bubbles up from the ground or where it has flowed from its source via a natural conduit. Such springs are the salvation of intrepid hikers and campers blazing new trails or following seldom-trod mountain paths. Other rustic bathing spots with no accommodations may be found near mountain villages or farming communities where local inhabitants have built a simple

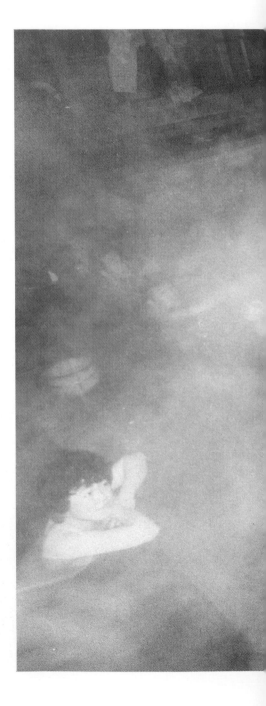

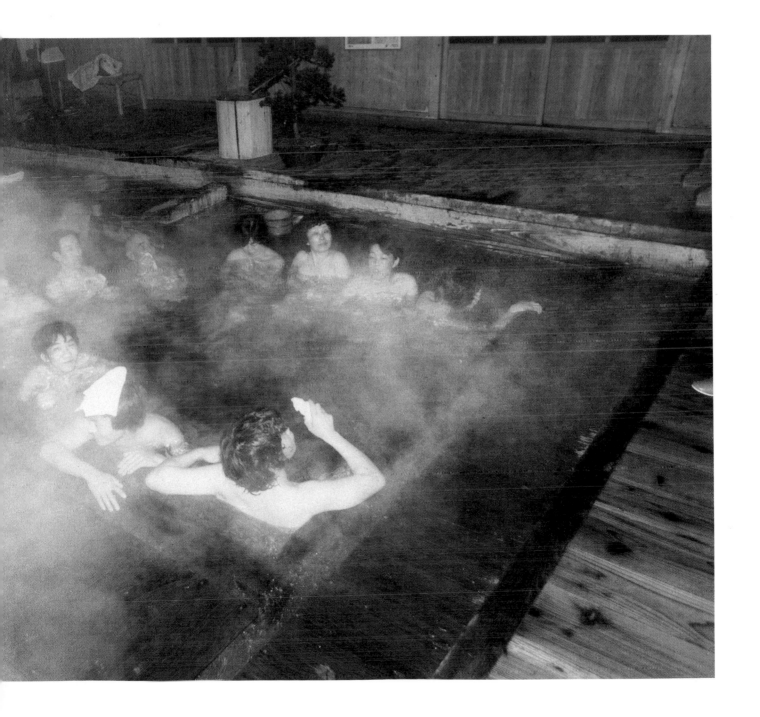

A single inn, the Chojukan, provides the sole accommodations at Hoshi hot spring. Its bathhouse, built late in the nineteenth century, combines the massive roof-beams of traditional Japanese farmhouses with delicately arched windows of a decidedly Victorian style.

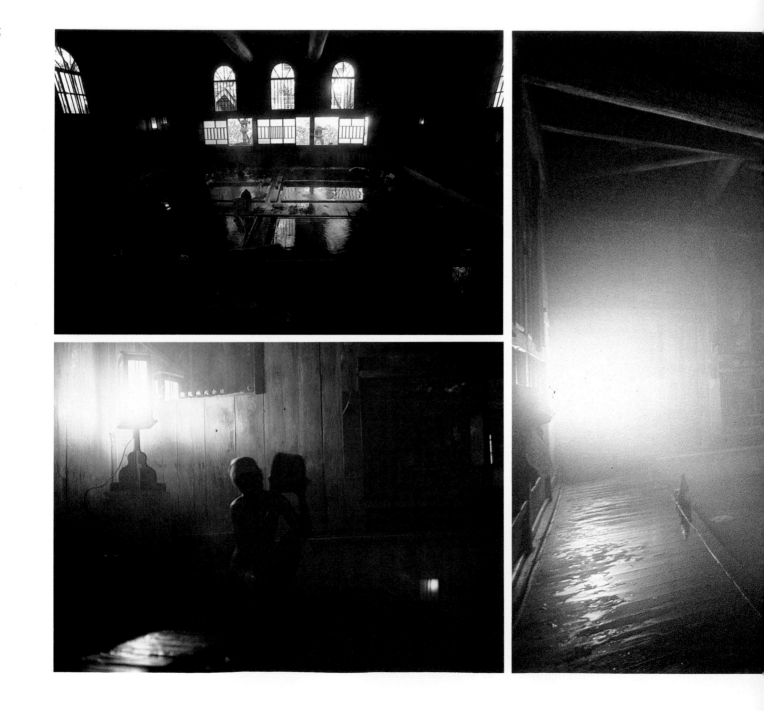

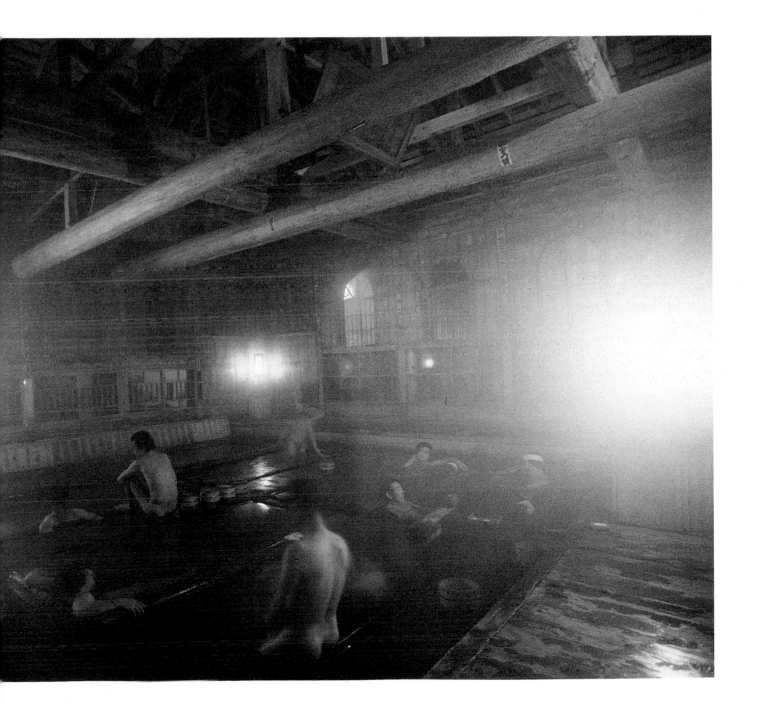

At this spring in Osawa, Iwate Prefecture, the hot water has been dammed right where it bubbles forth alongside a mountain river. Bathers delight in soaking outdoors in this leafy setting while listening to the birds and the river rushing past.

concrete enclosure to hold the hot water from a spring and, covering it with a rudimentary lean-to or thatched roof, have created a bathhouse to retire to after their daily labors. The traditional practice among poor farmers, unable to afford luxurious inns, is to recover from their strenuous labors in simple hostels known as *tojiba* ("bath-cure places"), where for a few pennies they can rent a room at a hot spring and where they are permitted to prepare their own food and tend to their own needs. The hot water flowing through these unpretentious bathing establishments is the same as that which, down the road or on the other side of the mountain, fills the great pools or hothouse "jungle baths" or lavish pleasure domes in resort towns.

A quick glance at a map of Japan reveals that some areas of the country are more richly endowed with hot springs than others. A cluster of town names printed in red, each accompanied by the familiar nationwide logo for *onsen*— three wavy lines representing steam rising from an encircling line indicating a pool—marks a concentration of hot springs. Hokkaido, Japan's northernmost island, shows such a cluster around Shikaribetsu in its central region, another around Niseko on its western coast, and another at Noboribetsu on the populous southern coast. But the red *onsen* mark is also sprinkled liberally all over the great, sparsely populated frontier that Hokkaido still represents in the Japanese mind. The most northern hot spring in the entire country is located at Wakkanai, separated by only a few miles of cold ocean water from Russian Sakhalin and the northern islands whose ownership Japan disputes with the Soviet Union.

The central mountains of northern Honshu are dense with thermal springs. On the map, some parts of Aomori, Iwate, Akita, Miyagi, Yamagata, and Fukushima prefectures are so crowded with springs that the otherwise pale-green map turns red. The same is true of the central regions of Honshu: Nagano Prefecture, roughly the size of Connecticut, has 140 hot-spring resorts; Niigata Prefecture, slightly smaller, has 93; and Gumma Prefecture, barely larger than the state of Delaware, has 63. For some reason, there are somewhat fewer hot

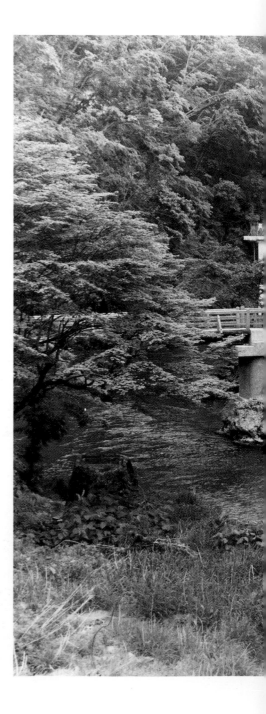

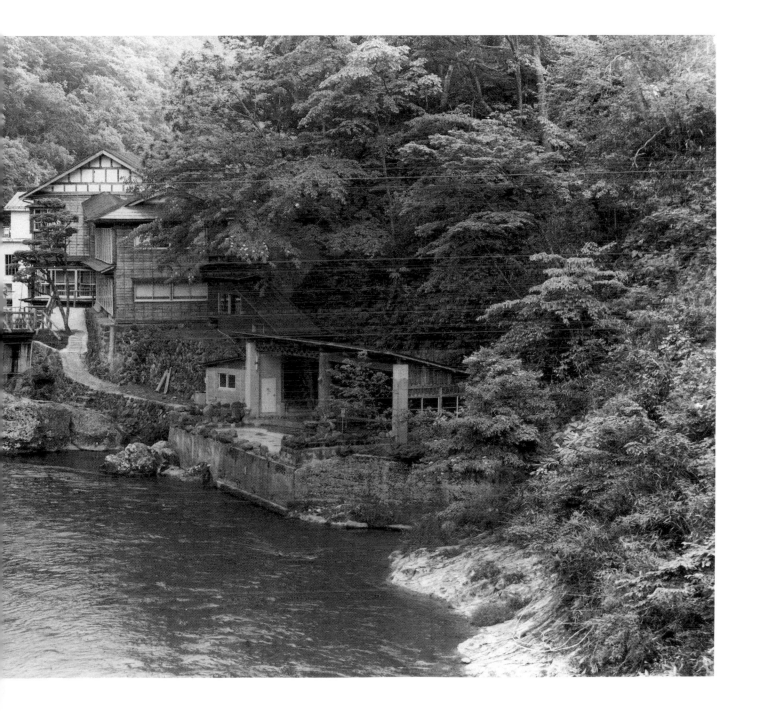

Bathing is at its best outdoors, in a *rotenburo*, where nature's heat warms the body and her scenic beauty refreshes the soul. The outdoor baths shown here include Osawa (*left, top and bottom*), Takaragawa (*right, top*), Noboribetsu (*right, bottom*), and Shuzenji (*far right*), where a bather luxuriates in the crystal-clear water of a *rotenburo*.

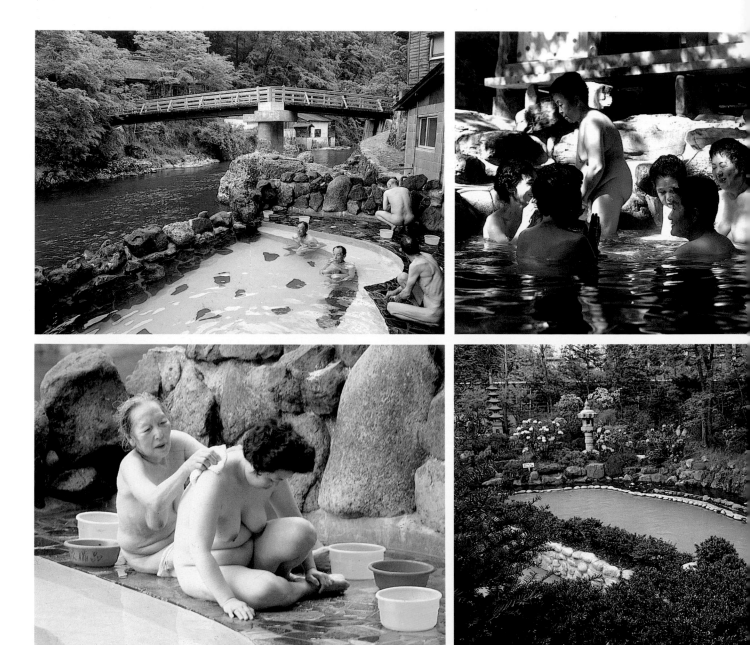

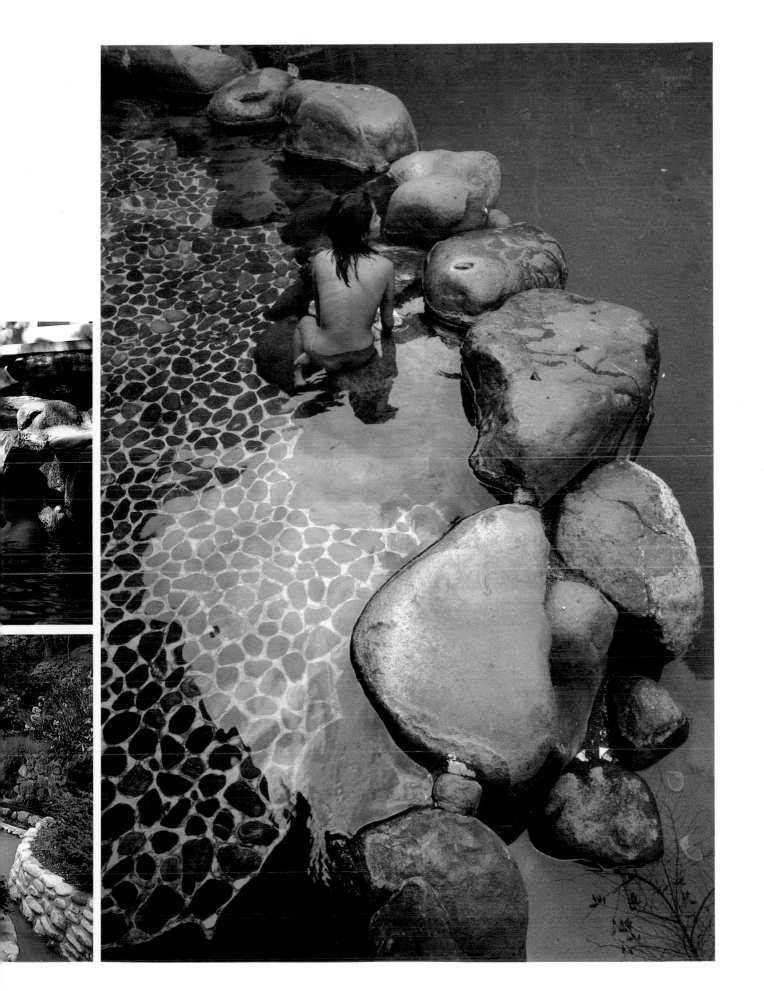

springs in the western half of Honshu, and relatively few on the island of Shikoku. Kyushu, however, at the southwest end of the chain of Japanese islands, is nearly as densely populated with hot springs as the north: the seven prefectures that make up Kyushu together possess nearly two hundred springs.

Although *onsen* are generally associated with scenic rural settings, they exist as well in Japan's cities. Tokyo, for example, has natural thermal springs at twenty-six different sites. The bathhouses built over them look much like the conventional public baths located all over the city, but they boast of restorative waters and charge an admission fee three to four times higher than the other bathhouses. The managers of city hot springs feel justified in charging more because, unlike public bathhouses, they receive no subsidy from the city government. A regular bathhouse is considered a necessity of social welfare whereas an *onsen,* by government standards, is a luxury and merits no special support.

In Japan, the mineral content of natural springs varies considerably from place to place, allowing local innkeepers to make extravagant claims about the unique healing powers of their waters. The hot springs of a single locality may be distinguished by a fairly consistent mineral content, or they may vary widely in composition. Beppu, for example, has hot springs of virtually every type found in Japan: sulphurous springs, alkaline springs, simple salt springs, acid springs, ferrous springs, and springs of high radium content. This variety accounts in large part, no doubt, for Beppu's enormous success as a resort and for its extraordinary density of hotels and inns (there are nearly 850 hostelries in the town proper, and hundreds more scattered about the surrounding mountains and villages).

Kusatsu, a popular hot-spring town about three hours north of Tokyo by train, has both intensely hot springs with a high sulphur content and cold springs so acidic that they are practically corrosive. The miraculous health-restoring properties of Kusatsu's waters have been widely known in Japan at least since the time of the first shogun, Minamoto no Yoritomo

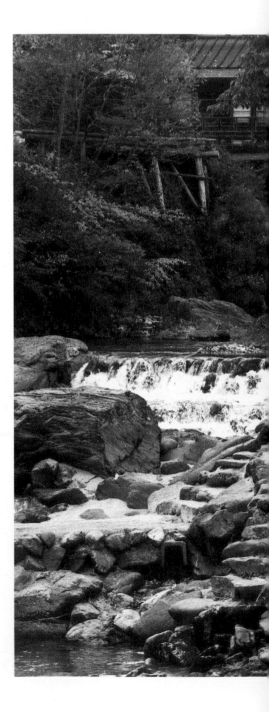

Takaragawa boasts one of the loveliest and most popular *rotenburo* in Japan. A series of rocky pools, brimming with hot water from natural springs, has been built alongside the cascading Takara River. Other pools are located upstream, beyond the changing room at the center of the photograph.

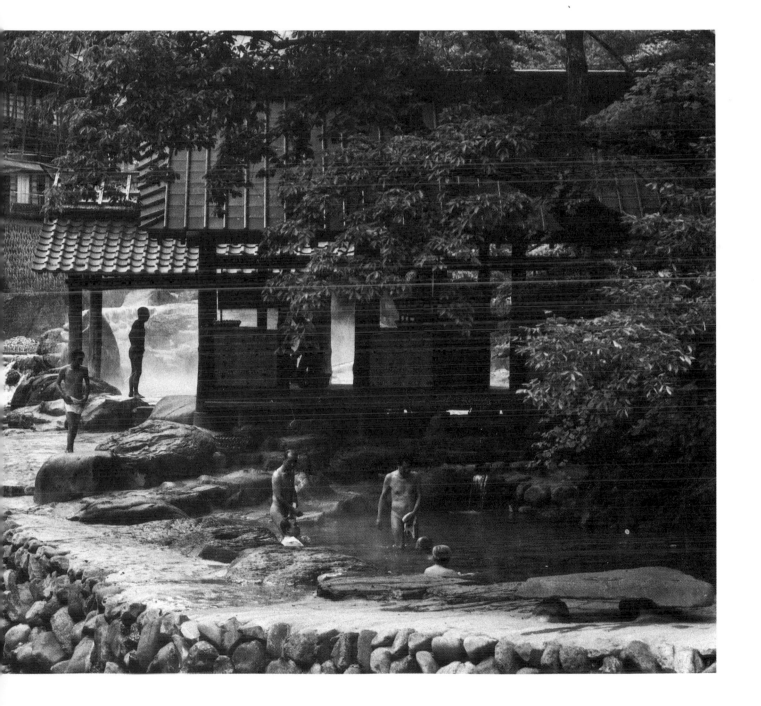

The great *rotenburo* at Takaragawa. Summer and winter, night and day, hot water bubbles into this open-air bath that is one of Japan's largest and most celebrated.

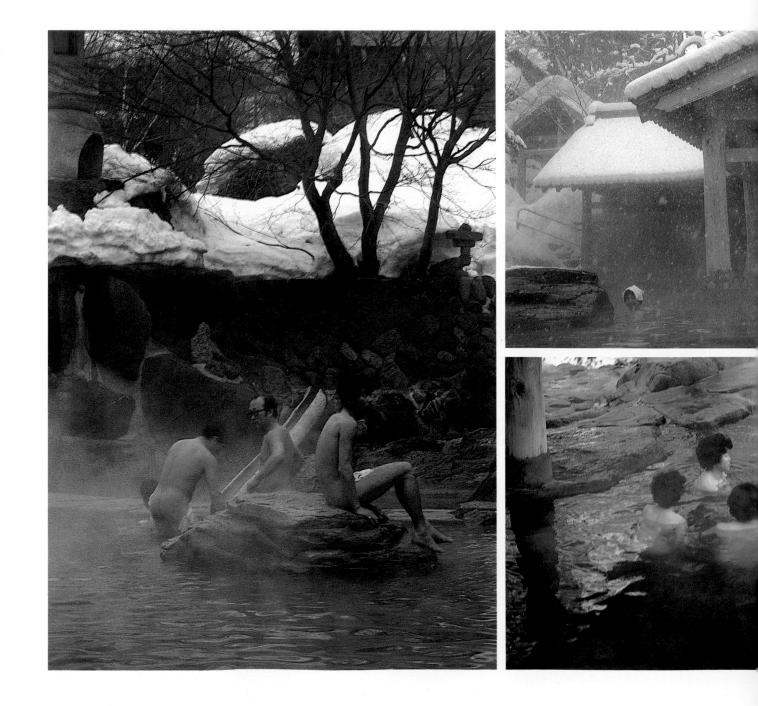

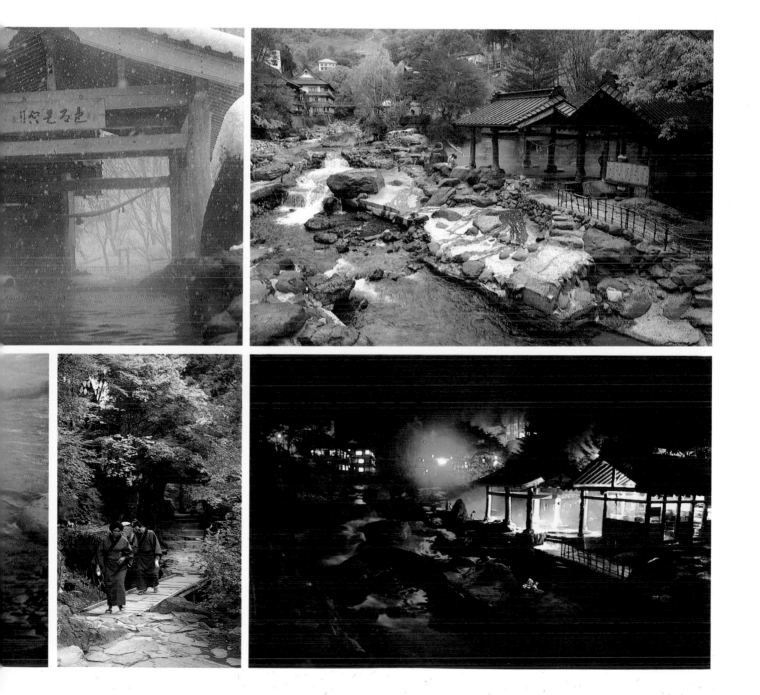

The penetrating warmth of
Takaragawa's hot springs protects
bathers from the cold of winter.

136 (1147–99), who visited the spa repeatedly during the twelfth
century. The medicinal value of Kusatsu's waters were given an
international reputation by the German physician Edwin Bälz
(1849–1927), who bathed there frequently and wrote about the
spa in several European medical journals. The temperature of
Kusatsu's hot springs ranges from 109° F to nearly 150° F (43°–
65° C), and the baths are kept so hot (between 120° F and 130° F)
that bathers can only tolerate them for a few minutes at a time.
An elaborate ceremony, a folk dance based on necessity, has
developed around the Kusatsu baths: a group of bathers stands
along a tub of scalding water as attendants reduce the temperature of the water by rhythmically stirring the slightly cooler
water from the bottom with long boards, singing as they work; at
a signal from the bathmaster, the bathers—as many as two hundred at a time—enter the painfully hot water and sit motionless
while the bathmaster calls out the number of remaining seconds
that they must endure this torture. It is unclear whether Dr.
Bälz's assertion that the Kusatsu baths would cure syphilis,
rheumatism, and chronic skin diseases was due to the chemical
properties of the water or the possibility that the diseases might
be boiled out of the sufferers. A local proverb claims that love is
the only grave disorder that Kusatsu cannot cure!

In Japan, as in Europe and America and every-
where else that hydrotherapy is practiced, the reliability and the
precise effect of certain waters on specific illnesses are matters
of unending controversy. That bathing in natural mineral
springs offers marvelously invigorating sensations is beyond
argument. *How* it works, however, is not. Quacks, charlatans,
and incredible claims abound in the imprecise science of
hydrotherapy. But no matter, since Japanese hot-spring enthu-
siasts—like their Occidental counterparts at White Sulphur
Springs in West Virginia, Bath in England, Baden-Baden in
Germany, or Carlsbad in Czechoslovakia—are drawn to these
resorts for recreational reasons as well. The treatments associated with certain springs in Japan have more often evolved
from folk tradition ("Saint So-and-so bathed here centuries ago
and imparted his miraculous healing powers to the water"),

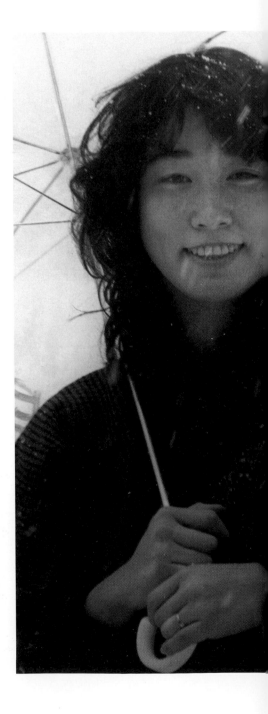

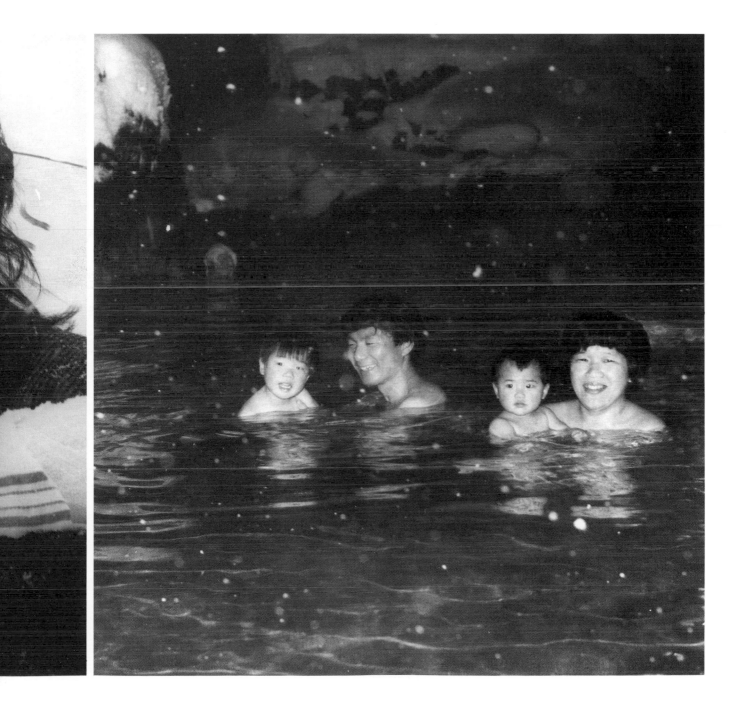

More scenes from Takaragawa.

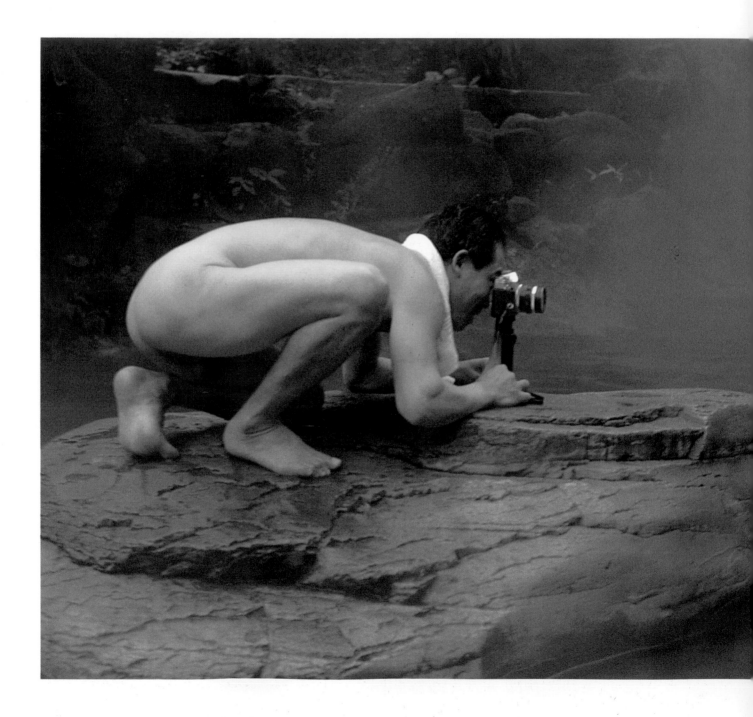

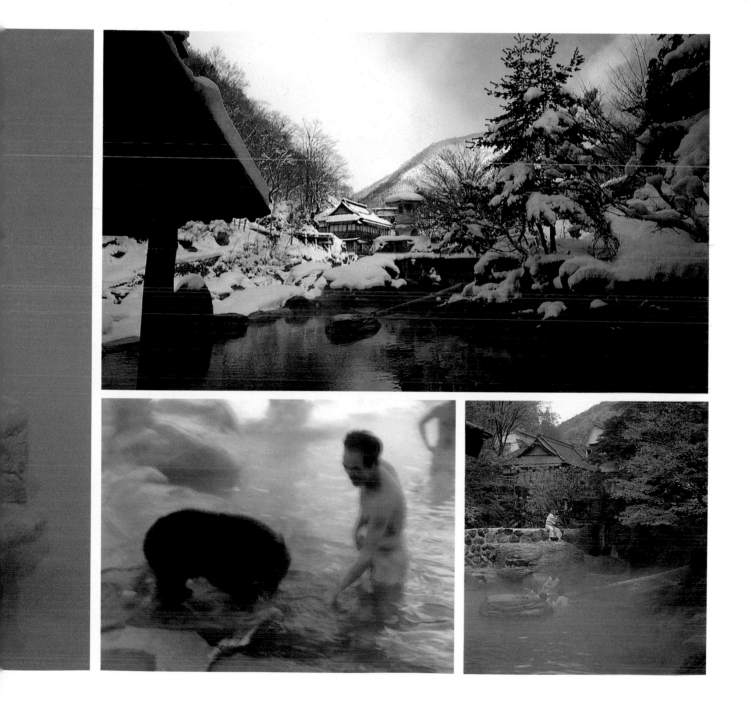

pseudohistorical legend ("Tokugawa Ieyasu's barren mistress bathed here for a week and immediately thereafter was able to conceive a child"), or simple local lore ("So-and-so's great-great-grandfather was cured of his rheumatism here") than from verifiable medical evidence. Nonetheless, the fact that such claims have persisted so long, surviving generation after generation of skeptics, is argument of a sort in support of the salutary effect the spring waters do seem to have on certain diseases. If nothing else, the very conviction that the mineral waters are helping to alleviate a condition of discomfort should markedly improve the bather's sense of well-being. The chart opposite provides a general survey of the types of hot springs that seem, according to widely accepted Japanese belief, to be efficacious in treating various afflictions.

On the wall of the dressing room of every hot-spring bath is a similar chart listing the mineral content of the water and the diseases it is supposed to cure or relieve. Most bathers never read these charts as they quickly shed their clothes and rush past into the bathroom. Those who do examine them will nod sagely as they read, and quickly forget the information as they slide comfortably into the warming waters of the tub.

Japanese people like their baths hot—very hot—and their volcanic land obliges them. In many hot springs the water flows out of the ground at temperatures well above the boiling point of 212° F (100° C). The average temperature of hot springs in Oita Prefecture, where Beppu is located, is 136° F (58° C), though at some springs in Beppu scalding water gushes forth at 233° F (112° C), and obviously must be cooled before bathers can enter it. At springs where the water emerges at a natural temperature of about 107.6° F (42° C), a perfectly comfortable level for most Western bathers, it usually must be heated artificially to suit the tastes of Japanese clientele, who prefer to bathe at temperatures between 110° F and 120° F. Many Westerners find Japanese bath temperatures, even at the low end of the spectrum, unbearably hot, though others, after some practice, claim they wouldn't want it any cooler.

Type of onsen:	As a bath— effective for:	As a drink— effective for:	Representative onsen:
Simple *onsen* (containing low level of mineral salts)	Neuralgia Rheumatism		Hakone Yumoto, Tonozawa, Kinugasa, Takaragawa
Carbon-dioxyated *onsen*	High blood pressure Heart disease Neuralgia	Dyspepsia Stomach catarrh Constipation	Arima, Ayukawa, Isobe
Earthy carbon-dioxyated *onsen*	Rheumatism Gout	Kidney stones Intestinal catarrh Diarrhea	Akakura, Nagayu
Sodium bicarbonate *onsen*	Burns Scars Skin diseases	Diabetes Glycosuria Pyelitis Bladder catarrh	Yunomine, Arima, Hirayu
Salt *onsen*	Sciatica Rheumatism	Anemia Lympha-denitis	Arima, Wakura, Atami, Yugawara, Miyanoshita
Sulphur-salt *onsen*	Rheumatism Neuralgia	Piles Nettle rash	Yamashiro, Kona, Izusan
Iron *onsen*	Neuralgia Rheumatism	Nervous debility Hysteria Sterility	Ikao, Beppu
Sulphur *onsen*	Skin diseases Rheumatism Diabetes Glycosuria	Diabetes Glycosuria Rheumatism Gout	Ashinoyu, Akakura
Alkaline *onsen*	Skin diseases Neuralgia		Murota, Kazawa
Acid *onsen*	Rheumatism VD Skin diseases		Kusatsu, Nasu Yumoto
Alum *onsen*	Rheumatism Skin diseases Nettle rash		Yunohanazawa, Myoban
Radium *onsen*	Neuralgia Rheumatism	Neuralgia Rheumatism Stomach and intestinal catarrh	Tomimasu, Ena, Ikeda

Based on a chart from *Sensual Water* by Bernard Barber and Dana Levy

The "Cave of Forgotten Return" at the Urashima Hotel in Katsuura. in this magical setting, the warm waters lull bathers into imagining themselves to be modern reincarnations of Urashima Taro, the legendary fisherman who discovered eternal youth in the watery realm of the Sea Dragon. Like Rip Van Winkle, Urashima Taro aged only when he woke from his enchanted dream and returned home decades after his disappearance.

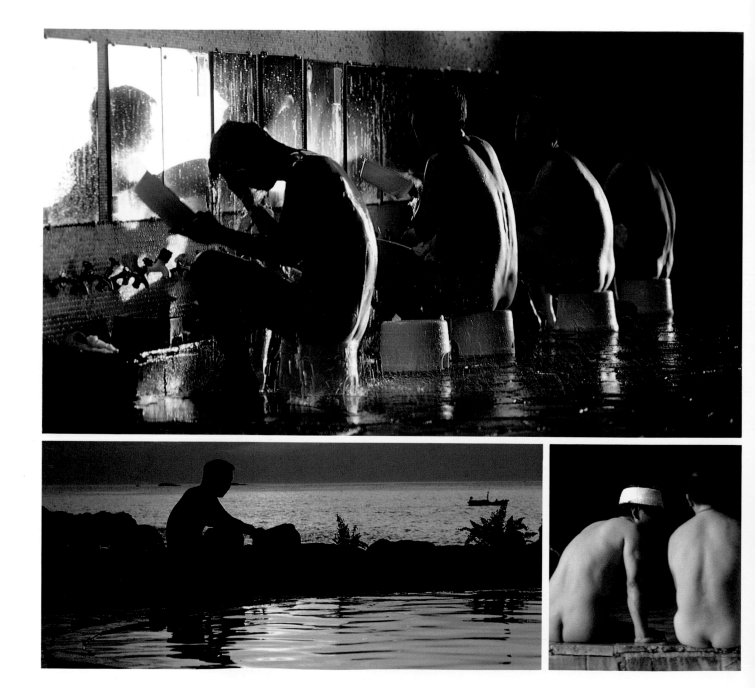

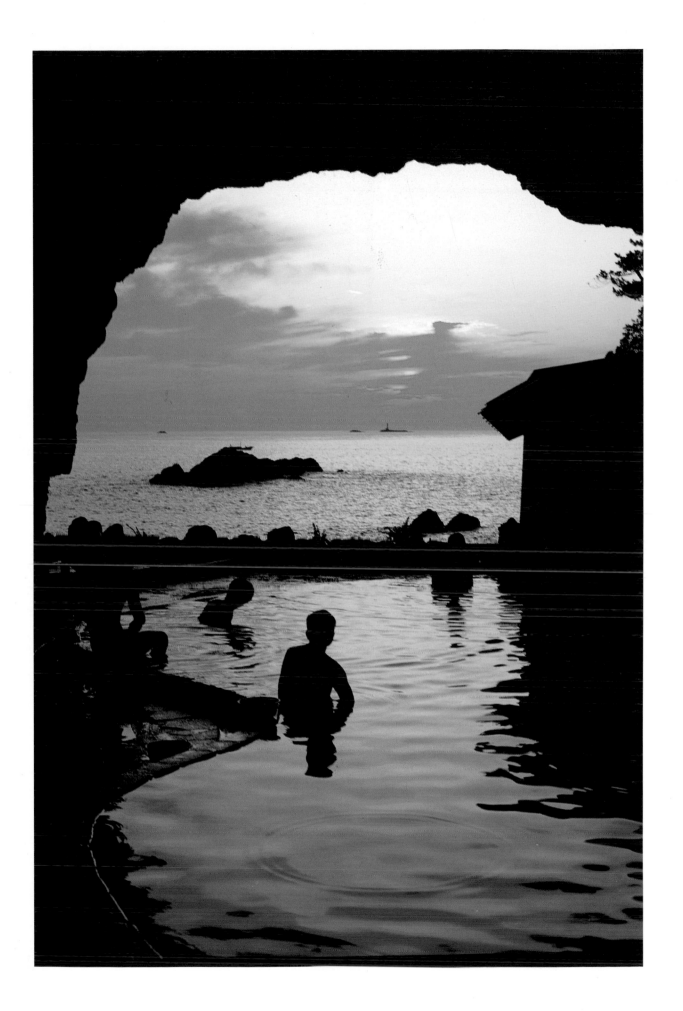

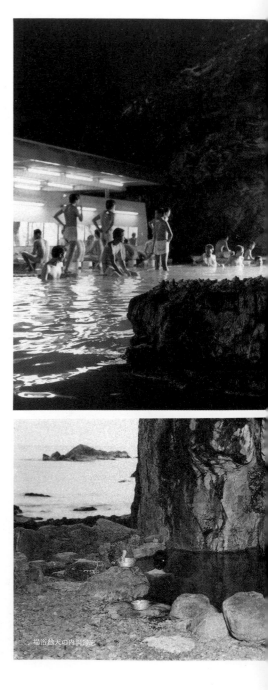

The fabled cave baths at Katsuura, where hot water from natural springs fills the pools in rocky grottoes before spilling into the sea.

Bathing at such hot temperatures carries some risk for people with high blood pressure and consequently should be of only short duration. The usual Japanese practice is to sit a few minutes in the scalding tub and then get out and cool off a bit before entering again. Doctors advise staying no longer than three minutes in water over 123° F (51° C) and avoiding hot baths immediately after meals. Even at somewhat lower temperatures, the gentle euphoria brought on by a hot Japanese bath can turn into a fainting spell if one soaks too long.

But at just the right temperature, in pleasant surroundings, and in agreeable company, Japanese hot-spring baths can seem close to paradise. Among the many Japanese writers who have tried to capture the ecstasy of the bath is Natsume Soseki, who describes it beautifully in this passage from his 1906 novel *Kusamakura* (literally, "pillow of grass"):

> Brr! It was cold. Towel in hand, I went down for a warm bath. I undressed in a small matted room and then went down the four steps into the bathroom which was about twelve feet square. There appeared to be no shortage of stones in these parts, for both the floor and the lining of the sunken bath tank in the centre were of pebbles set in cement. The tank was about the size of the vats they used to make bean-curd, being roughly four feet deep. This place was called a mineral spring, so there were presumably many mineral ingredients in the water. As, in spite of this, it was clear and transparent, I found it very pleasant to bathe in. From time to time some of the water found its way into my mouth, but it had no distinctive taste or odour. This spring was said to have medical properties, but I never took the trouble to find out what ailments it was supposed to cure. Since I myself was not suffering from any illness the idea that the spring might have any practical value did not enter my head. As I stepped into the tank, all I was thinking of was a poem by the Chinese poet Po Chü-i that expresses the feeling of pleasure which the mere mention of the word "hotspring" rouses in me.

> The waters of the spring caress;
> And smooth away all coarseness from my skin.

All that I ask of any hot spring is that it give me just such a pleas-

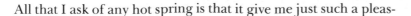

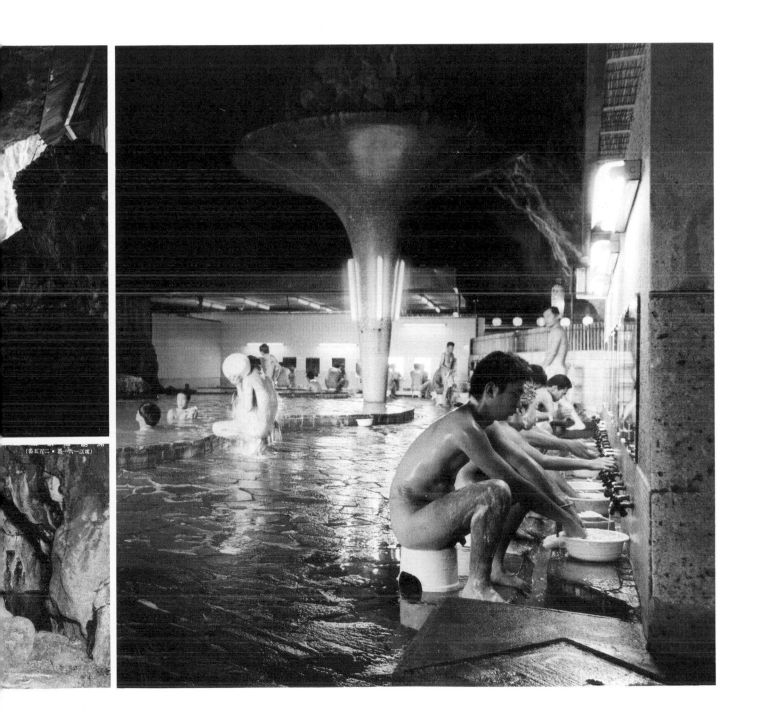

（番五花二・番一六一話電）

"Jungle baths" create another kind of magic: Is one indoors or out? In Japan or on some distant tropical isle? Or simply in paradise? In these fantasy realms, bathers forget everyday cares and cast off all restraints. Anything seems possible in these watery wonderlands.

146

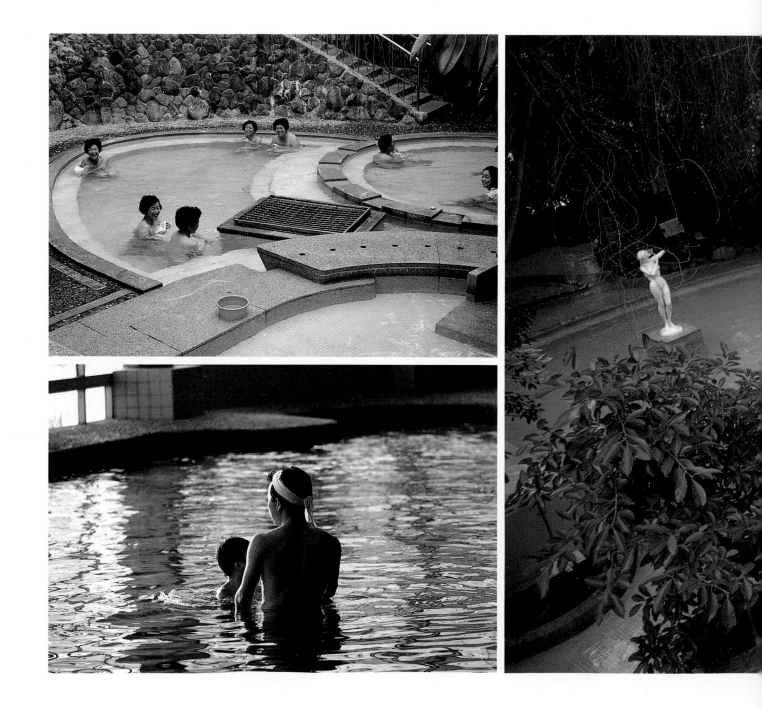

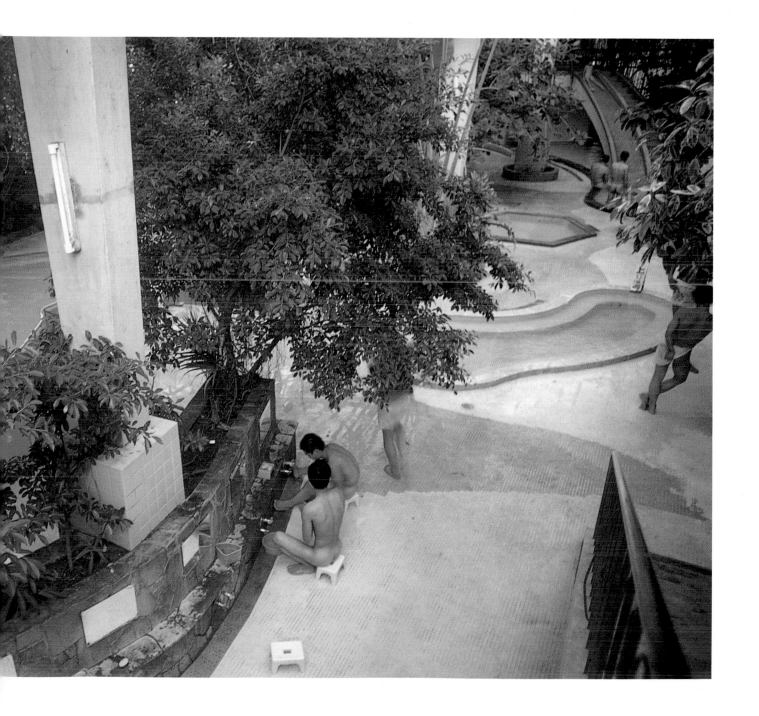

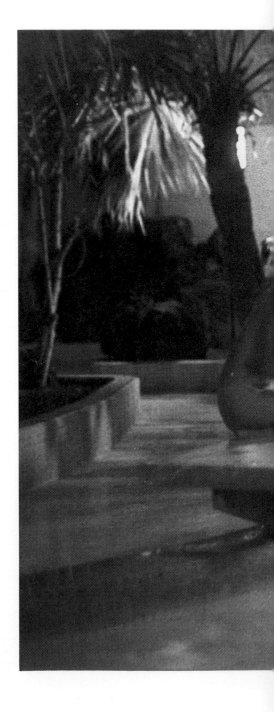

Laughter echoes through the great "jungle bath" at Ibusuki. Behind this group of high-spirited women, a younger bather enjoys the thrill of a water slide into another pool of steamy water.

ant feeling, but if it is unable to do so, in my opinion it is worthless.

The water came up to my chest, and I sat there soaking myself in it thoroughly. I do not know from where the hot water gushed, but it was constantly pouring over the sides in an attractive stream. I was happy, and very much at ease as there in the springtime I felt beneath my feet the warmth of those stones which were never dry....

...there are many things which can charm me, and whose cry finds an answering echo within me; but only on a spring evening, with my body softly enveloped in clouds of steam from a hot bath, can I feel that I belong to a bygone age. The steam which draped itself around me was not so dense that I was unable to see. Nor yet was it as thin as a layer of sheer silk which may easily be torn aside to reveal the ordinary mortal figure beneath. I was isolated in a warm rainbow: shut in on all sides by steam from which I could never emerge however many layers I might pull aside. One can talk of becoming drunk on wine, but I have never heard the phrase "to become drunk on vapour." Even if there were such a phrase, it could not of course be used of mist, and is rather too strong to use of haze. Nevertheless, it does become apt when used to describe the steam rising from a hot bath, but then only in the context of a spring evening.

Leaning my head back against the side of the tank, I let my weightless body rise up through the hot water to the point of least resistance. As I did so I felt my soul to be floating like a jellyfish. The world is an easy place to live in when you feel like this. You throw off the bars of desire and physical attachment. Lying in the hot water, you allow it to do with you as it likes, and become absorbed into it. The more freely you are able to float, the easier life becomes, until if your very soul floats, you will be in a state more blessed than had you become a disciple of Christ....

Soseki's protagonist in *Kusamakura* is a painter, who travels alone seeking spiritual revitalization and inspiration for his art. While it is not unheard of today for individuals seeking solitude to visit hot springs, they are the exceptions to the rule. Innkeepers are traditionally wary of solitary travelers, particularly lone women, fearing that their objective is suicide. Indeed, hot springs have traditionally been favorite spots for

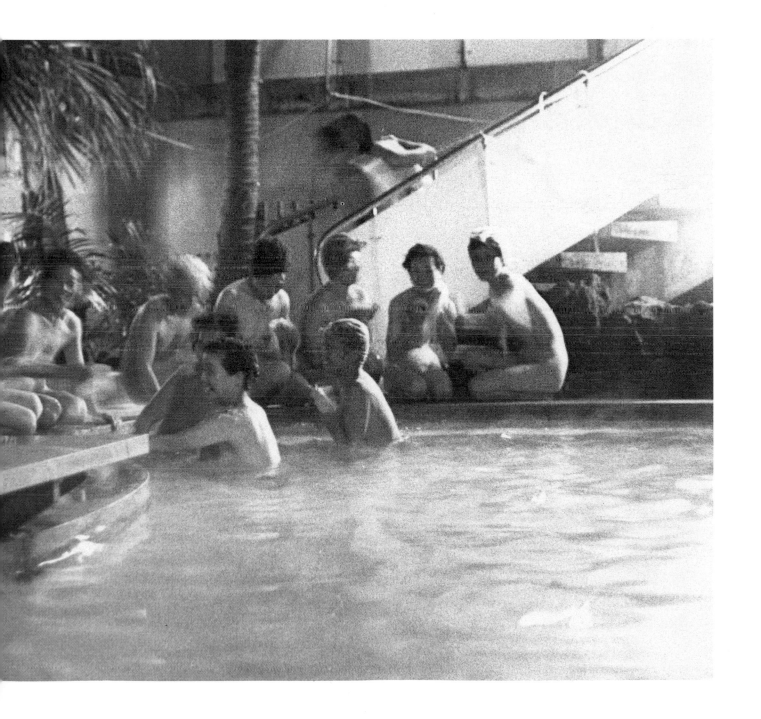

Japan's hot springs are not restricted exclusively to human bathers. Indeed, many springs were originally discovered by hunters tracking injured animals, which nursed their wounds in the soothing warm waters of natural springs.

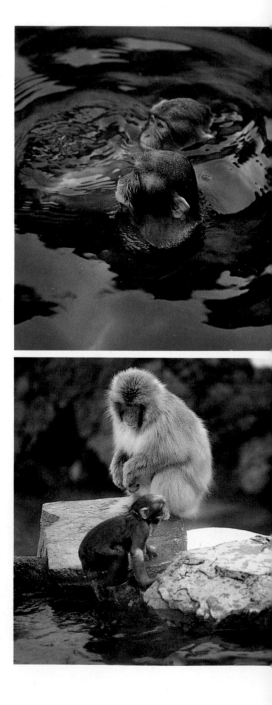

150   suicides, especially the double suicides of ill-fated lovers, because of their beautiful natural settings and their romantic, often somewhat erotic, atmosphere. Hot-spring resorts are detached from the realities of everyday life, separated from the associations that bind an individual to family and home and work, and it is in such places that he or she is emboldened to express true feelings, including self-destructive ones. Japanese film directors and novelists fill their works with scenes set at hot springs, cherishing no doubt the pathetic ironies that contrast the torment of a despairing individual with the general merriment that enlivens the place.

For the most part, Japanese pleasure seekers flock to *onsen* in groups, the smallest group being two individuals—lovers, honeymooners, an elderly married couple, a businessman and his young mistress—and the largest group being a mass gathering of people sharing some common interest. An entire class of high-school students, scores of giggling girls and self-consciously boisterous adolescent boys, may take a field trip to a hot spring that has some special historical significance; teachers accompanying the group point out the local historical remains and struggle to maintain order, while the kids frisk noisily about in the hot-spring pools. Or a typical group might be the members of a rural farm cooperative, enjoying an autumn outing after their labors of bringing in the harvest. Or it might be a company party: one department of a large firm or an entire small company—bosses, white-collar workers, and secretaries all together—enjoying a respite from the tedium of daily office activities. Or a group of middle-aged housewives, all of them aspiring poets who are taking a writing course together at one of the "culture centers" that have sprung up recently in many urban communities. Or an outing led by the *madamu* of a bar or nightclub, treating her bartenders and hostesses to a weekend off and joined by a select assemblage of favorite regular customers. Or the entire faculty of a local school, ostensibly on a retreat to plan the year's curriculum.

The composition of a group outing can be as varied as Japanese society itself, and excuses for taking a trip

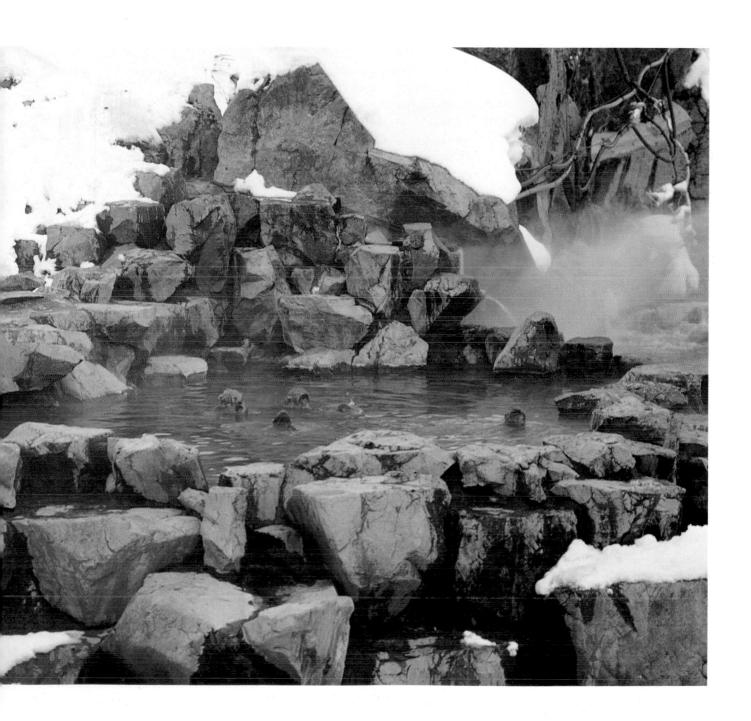

152   together are never hard to come by. Every Japanese is a member, in the course of his lifetime, of several important circles of associates—first his immediate family, later his school classmates, club members, co-workers, fellow hobbyists, and the like. He is rarely completely alone, and much of his identity is derived from his membership in the group. These circles of friends, colleagues, or associates are loosely termed *nakama,* a word that can be translated simply as group or company of friends, but which connotes a fellowship of shared sensibilities and identities. Within such circles of *nakama,* a typical Japanese person feels comfortable, accepted, at home; apart from them, he is lost, adrift in a sea of strangers, alienated and bewildered. An individual is always part of several *nakama,* sometimes interlocking circles, sometimes widely separated by time, space, or attitude, and with each of them he shares a part of his personality.

      The purpose of group excursions to hot-spring resorts is, primarily, to revitalize and deepen one's sense of *nakama.* It is an unspoken objective, of course, for the ostensible reasons are sightseeing, rest, and the fun of sampling new mineral springs. But underlying everything is the urge to share experience and to reconfirm one's membership in a particular fraternity.

      Onsen are perfectly equipped to fulfill this purpose, for what better way to reaffirm a sense of intimacy can there be than for friends to bathe together, make merry together, and sleep together? *Onsen* hotels can accommodate groups of any size—from the small nuclear family to gatherings of several hundred people. They arrive at the resort, immediately shed their clothes, and with them all attachments to the society they have left behind at home, and don identical *yukata* (light cotton kimono) and robes supplied by the hotel. Throughout their stay, whether enjoying the entertainment provided by the establishment or wandering through the town sightseeing or shopping for souvenirs, they wear the same comfortable "uniform," reveling in their sense of togetherness.

      To a Westerner, concerned with personal identity and individuality, this might represent a loss of self. The

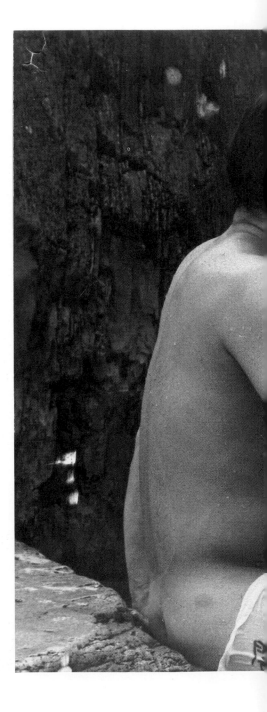

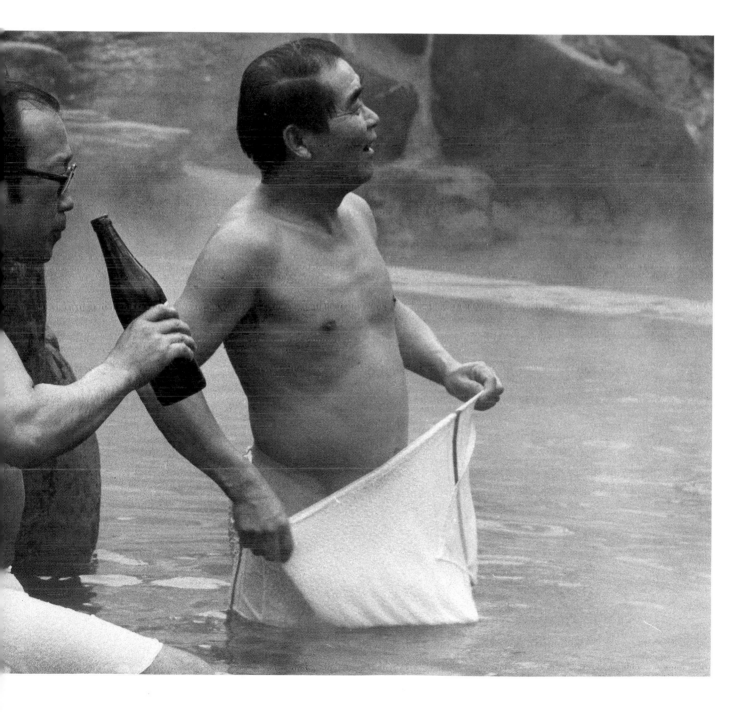

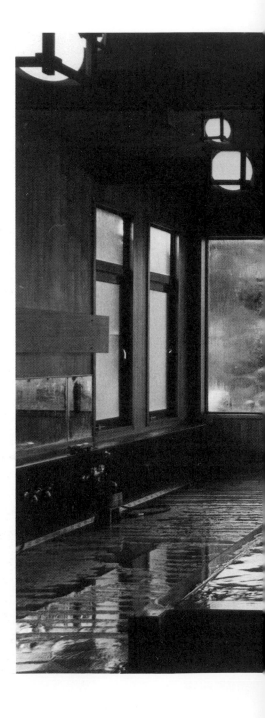

A quiet moment in a bath at the Shuzenji hot-spring resort in Izu. The entire room, including the huge tub, is built of aromatic *hinoki* wood.

154 Japanese, however, see the community of spirit represented by group activity only in a positive light: the individual is bolstered and reassured by interaction with close comrades, personality flowers when nurtured by the appropriate *nakama,* and the achievements of the group are improved when the talents of each member are merged with those of his companions.

Since baths are the principal attraction of *onsen* resorts, a large section of the inn or hotel is given over to bathrooms. Many guest rooms or suites these days have their own attached baths, but these are small and cramped, designed for no more than two people to use at a time. Far more pleasurable are the large common baths downstairs. There, visitors can enjoy a spaciousness unavailable to them at home and the company of their own group or of other guests of the hotel.

Divided into men's bath and women's bath, with the men's usually having the edge in size, the common baths occupy the most choice location in the hotel, comparable to the grand ballroom or main dining room of a Western resort hotel. Unlike the small, clinical bathing cubicles of most mineral-spring health resorts in the West, however, such baths may be shared by as many as sixty or seventy people at once. Since all washing, shampooing, and rinsing is done outside the main tank or pool, at faucets arranged along the sides of the room, no soap ever enters the pool. Bathers soak in clean, naturally hot water that is constantly being replenished from the source of the spring. These large bathrooms command the finest view of the landscape surrounding the hotel, and are easily accessible from all parts of the building. Usually they are on the ground floor, and if the hotel doesn't overlook a broad vista of mountains or seacoast, the baths may open onto a picturesque garden, satisfying the traditional requirement that life should be lived in close relationship to nature. Weather permitting, large sliding-glass doors between the bathroom and garden are opened, and often the bathing pool, which is actually indoors, is separated from a garden pond by only a thin wall, furthering the sensation that the space is continuous with the garden outside.

Bathing in the open air is perhaps the most

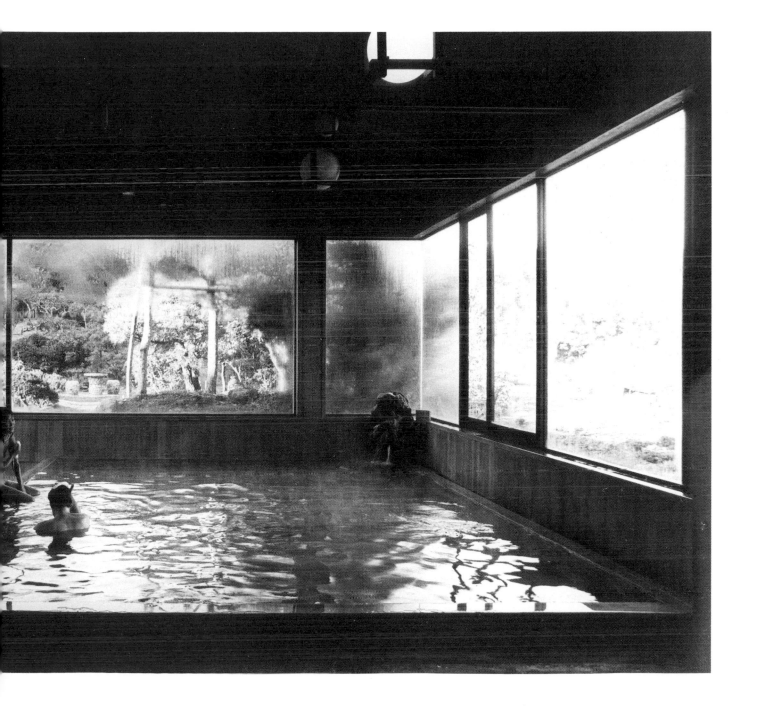

Going through the elaborately carved gateway to the Dogo hot-spring bath-house in Matsuyama City, the visitor passes several centuries back in time to the Edo period. Under the roof of this large building are several bathhouses, which draw on the waters of three different hot springs. The building and its baths provided the setting for part of Natsume Soseki's beloved comic novel *Botchan*.

pleasurable feature of many hot-spring hotels. In outdoor pools, known as *rotenburo*, one comes closest to a primal communion with nature that surely must remain somewhere deep in our subconscious memories. The term *rotenburo*, literally "a bath amid the dew under an open sky," captures the exquisitely lyrical sensation of this type of bath, where naked, immersed in clear hot water, one is exposed to the sky or stars overhead. Another attraction of *rotenburo* is that the social inhibitions regarding gender are often forgotten. While most Japanese hot-spring hotels today separate the sexes in their indoor baths, such distinctions are literally thrown to the winds in the outdoor pools where men and women frequently bathe together. Even where separate *rotenburo* are provided for men and women, they are usually separated by little more than a few rocks or bushes, and there tends to be a great deal of crossing back and forth.

Originally, *rotenburo* were located right at the source of a spring, a rock-girded pool that formed naturally where the hot water bubbled up from a fissure in the earth. In earlier times it was a particularly fortunate inn that could offer its guests a garden *rotenburo* as well as an indoor bath. Today, the pleasures of *rotenburo* bathing have become so popular (several Japanese magazines are devoted exclusively to them and there is a popular television program that features a different one each week) that many inns have created them: even inns hemmed in by other buildings in crowded towns have managed to transform their small gardens into *rotenburo* by excavating a pool, lining its bottom with small pebbles and its sides with boulders, piping in hot water from a hot spring and planting greenery in artful arrangements to simulate a natural pool in a forested glen. Great natural *rotenburo,* such as those at Takaragawa in Gumma Prefecture, Sakunami in Miyagi, and Ogawa in Toyama, to mention only a few, attract crowds in all seasons: in winter, with snowdrifts surrounding the steaming outdoor pool, bathing takes on a special excitement; the rest of the year, one soaks amid chirping birds in a leafy bower of striking natural beauty.

Another recent fad is the attempt by large hotels to simulate exotic tropical environments in indoor bathing

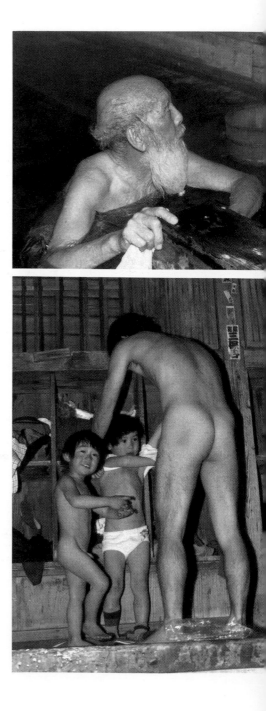

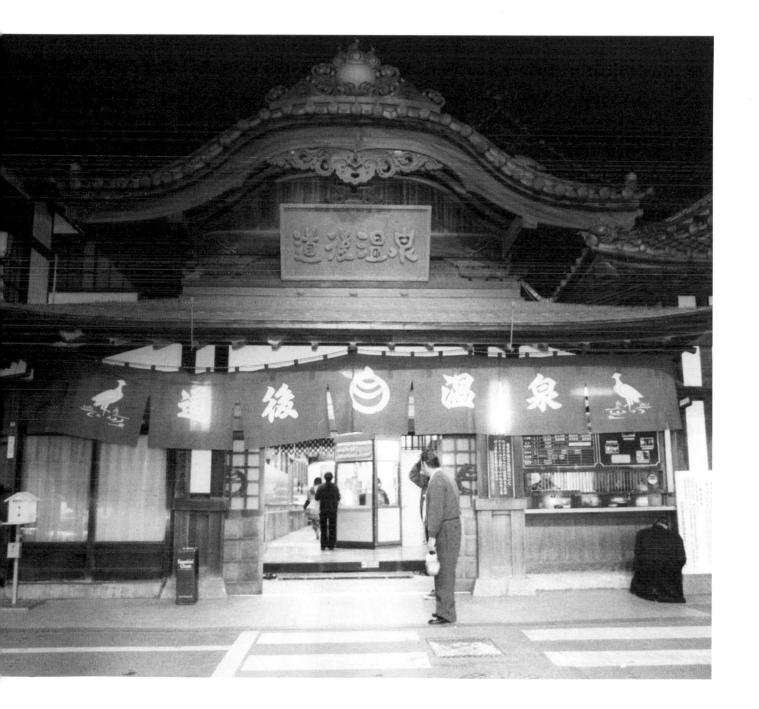

The *onsen* spirit engenders marvelous flights of fancy. For bathers who delight in immersing themselves in hot-spring waters and in simultaneously taking in the superb views of a rocky coast, the gondola baths of Arita provide a soaring experience. In an indoor bath at the same resort (*lower left*), hot water flows from a giant *sakè* bottle, splashing first into an oversized *sakè* cup and then into the bathing pool.

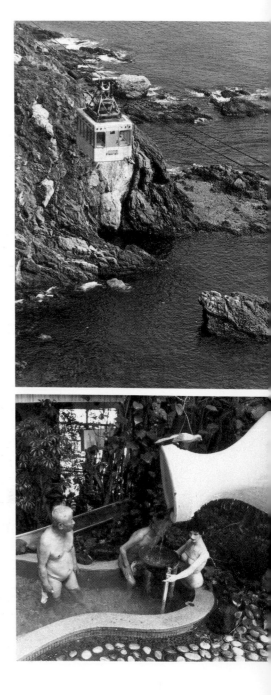

pavilions. Called "jungle baths," they have delighted visitors at large spa towns like Atami, Ibusuki, Beppu, and Noboribetsu. Within giant glass hothouses, often constructed on hotel rooftops, are built tiled hot-spring pools surrounded by tropical ferns and vines, hibiscuses, bougainvilleas, and many varieties of palm trees, all of which thrive in the warm humid atmosphere. Basking in the pools, bathers imagine themselves on the beaches or in the jungles of island paradises in the South Seas. Further elaborating on the jungle baths, perhaps taking inspiration from Disneyland, some enterprising hotel managers have developed "theme baths" with environments designed to look like underwater grottoes or even futuristic "Star Wars" settings. These fantasy worlds appeal no less to parents than to their excited children. Amid these exotic surroundings are bathing pools every bit as fantastic: in addition to the regular hot-spring baths are pools filled with milk, mud, water of especially high sulphur content, sand, even warm damp coffee beans. The adventurous bather moves from one substance to the next, showering between each tub, his body soaking in the medicinal, aphrodisiacal, or restorative properties of each.

When set free in the hedonistic atmosphere of a hot-spring resort, the Japanese fervor for novelty and exoticism knows no bounds. Some of its more extreme manifestations are baths with glass bottoms set in a river so bathers can watch fish swimming beneath them, funicular baths with tubs in glass-walled gondolas that allow bathers to take in scenic views as they swing in ropeways high in the air, and even a solid-gold bathtub in which *onsen* addicts are allowed to soak for an exorbitant fee. Clearly, with the ingenuity of the Japanese, coupled with their passion for bathing, the possibilities are endless!

Another major attraction of hot-spring resorts, in addition to the waters and the scenic or historical sights, is the food. So important is it that advertisements for resort hotels invariably picture colorful feasts alongside inviting views of the baths. Japanese inns and hotels, just like those at Hot Springs, Virginia, or Marienbad or Carlsbad, vie with one another in preparing lavish meals. In addition to a splendid array of fresh

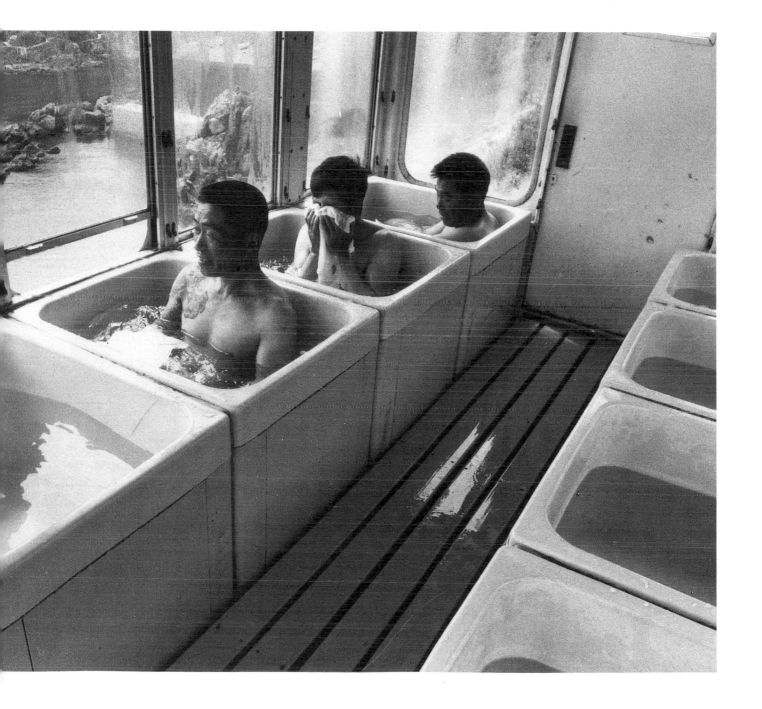

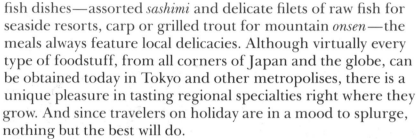

Along with the pleasures of hot-spring bathing, *onsen* resorts offer a wide variety of other amusements and entertainment, from game parlors to lavish meals.

fish dishes—assorted *sashimi* and delicate filets of raw fish for seaside resorts, carp or grilled trout for mountain *onsen*—the meals always feature local delicacies. Although virtually every type of foodstuff, from all corners of Japan and the globe, can be obtained today in Tokyo and other metropolises, there is a unique pleasure in tasting regional specialties right where they grow. And since travelers on holiday are in a mood to splurge, nothing but the best will do.

The mood generated by the *onsen* experience is one of innocent hedonism. The baths prepare body and spirit for sensual pleasures, and the meals and ample liquid refreshment delight both the eye and tongue. Freed from the customary restraints of everyday life and from the hard work that is their usual routine, hot-spring patrons are in holiday spirits, and for their after-hours amusement the resorts offer numerous attractions. The largest hotels have nightclubs, theaters, shopping arcades, video parlors, and a seemingly endless array of other enticements all under the same roof. In smaller establishments and in more old-fashioned hot-spring towns, pleasure seekers must leave their inns to find entertainment. Laughing and singing as they parade up and down the main streets and back alleys of the town, all dressed alike in robes provided by their inn (and prominently displaying the name of the inn or design motifs identifying it), they find their way to bars and small nightclubs, vaudeville shows, mahjong or gambling parlors, striptease salons, and carnival arcades. *Onsen* geisha and prostitutes are ready to be of service, and feeling invigorated for the moment, revelers young and old set off in high spirits for a night on the town. But the hot baths and the lavish food and drink usually take their toll. Except on major holidays, when the partying can go on all night, most *onsen* towns, even the most bawdy of them, are quiet and closed up for the night long before midnight.

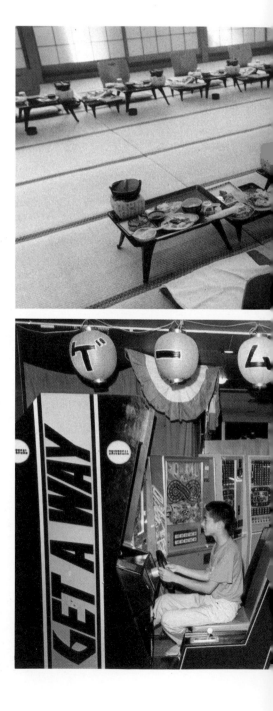

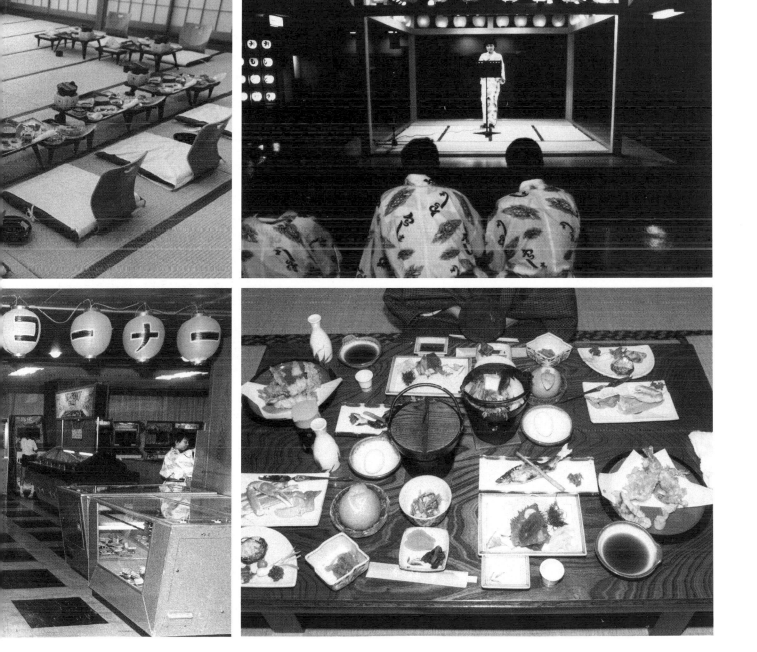

The baths at some of Japan's most famous hot-spring resorts. *Top, left to right:* Noboribetsu in Hokkaido, Beppu in Kyushu, and two small old-fashioned baths at Izu inns made famous as the settings of *The Izu Dancer*, a novella by the Nobel prizewinner Yasunari Kawabata. *Bottom, left to right:* baths at Osawa, Kusatsu, Osawa, and Hiratanai.

162

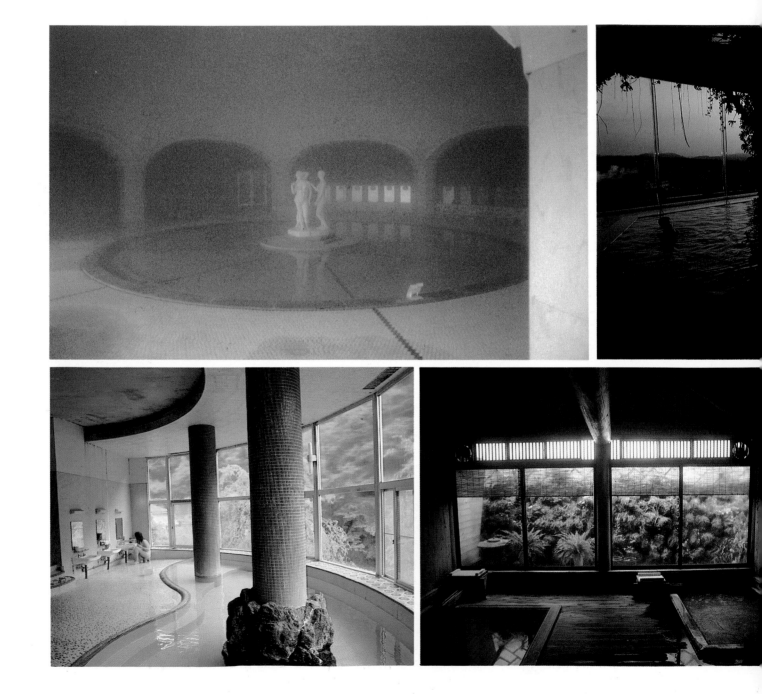

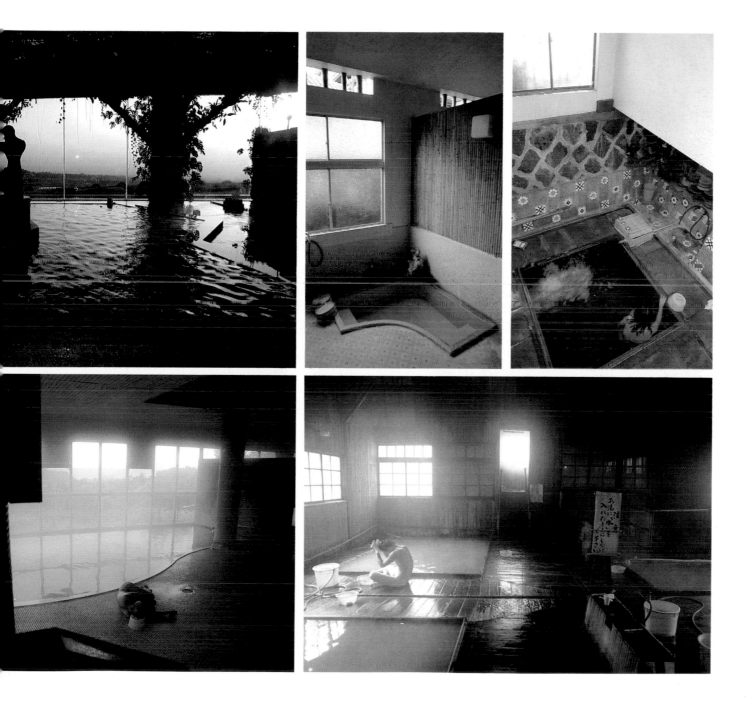

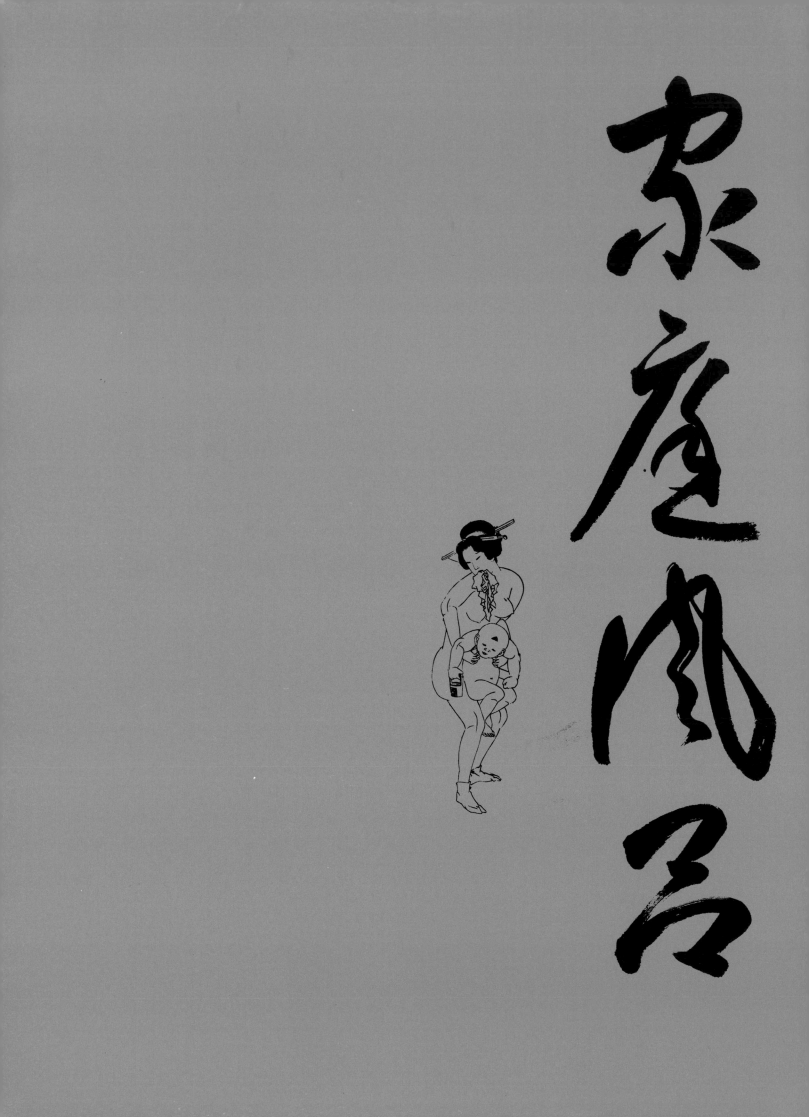

CHAPTER FIVE

The Domestic Bath

Bathing at home in Japan shares all the features of bathing out at public bathhouses or hot springs, except the company of others. The domestic tub, designed for a single individual or two at most, is just as deep and the water as hot. Japanese bathers would no more take a bar of soap into their tubs at home than they would in a public bath. The same process is followed in bathing, whether one does it in a public setting or alone at home: *before* entering the tub, one scrubs the body clean; next, one rinses away the soap and remaining grime; then, and only then—after the body is sparkling clean—one slips into the deep, clear hot water.

One of the greatest revolutions in domestic Japanese architecture in recent years has been the dramatic increase in bathing facilities and modern indoor plumbing. A mere two or three decades ago, the average new home built for a middle-class family generally did not include a bath. Toilet facilities were provided, even with modern plumbing (which only another decade or two earlier would have been a rarity), but a separate room for bathing was not necessarily part of the master plan. Public bathhouses were always within easy walking dis-

166 tance, after all, and a private bath was considered a special luxury. Wealthy homes possessed them, as they had for centuries. But the dwellers in modest family homes or apartments had to remain content—indeed, they often preferred—to stroll out of the house to take a bath several blocks away.

All of that has changed with remarkable speed. Today, virtually every private dwelling is built with a bath. Even modest apartments of only two rooms or so usually come equipped with a tiny, closet-size bathroom. Some, in fact, are one-piece molded plastic units designed specifically to fit inside the standard-size closet. With the popularization of domestic baths (and the simultaneous decline in the number of public bathing establishments) has come an explosion in new types of tubs and bath equipment.

The oldest bathtub on record in Japan is a rectangular wooden receptacle measuring 68 inches long, 33 inches wide, and 22 inches deep. From its shape, that of ancient Japanese ships, came the word for bathtub—*yubune,* or "hot-water ship." Although the first tubs were filled with hot water bucketful by bucketful, various means of heating the water in the tub were developed. By the late 1800s a variety of styles were in use, including a barrel-shaped vessel particularly popular among the citizenry of Edo. Most tubs were crafted of wood—Japanese cypress, cryptomeria, chestnut, Chinese black pine—or occasionally iron, and were heated simply by burning wood or charcoal beneath them. Edward Sylvester Morse, an American scientist invited in 1877 to teach at the Imperial University in Tokyo, describes them well in his book *Japanese Homes and Their Surroundings:*

> There are many forms of bathing-tubs, all of them being large and deep. Means for applying the heat direct, which is of course the most economical, is attained in various ways. In the common form, a small chamber of copper is introduced at one end near the bottom of the tub,—the mouth having a frame of stone or of clay or plaster. In this chamber a fire is built, and the water can be brought, if necessary, to the boiling point. Within the tub a few transverse bars prevent the bather from coming in contact with

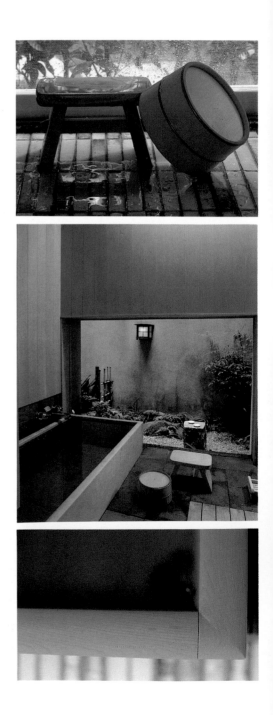

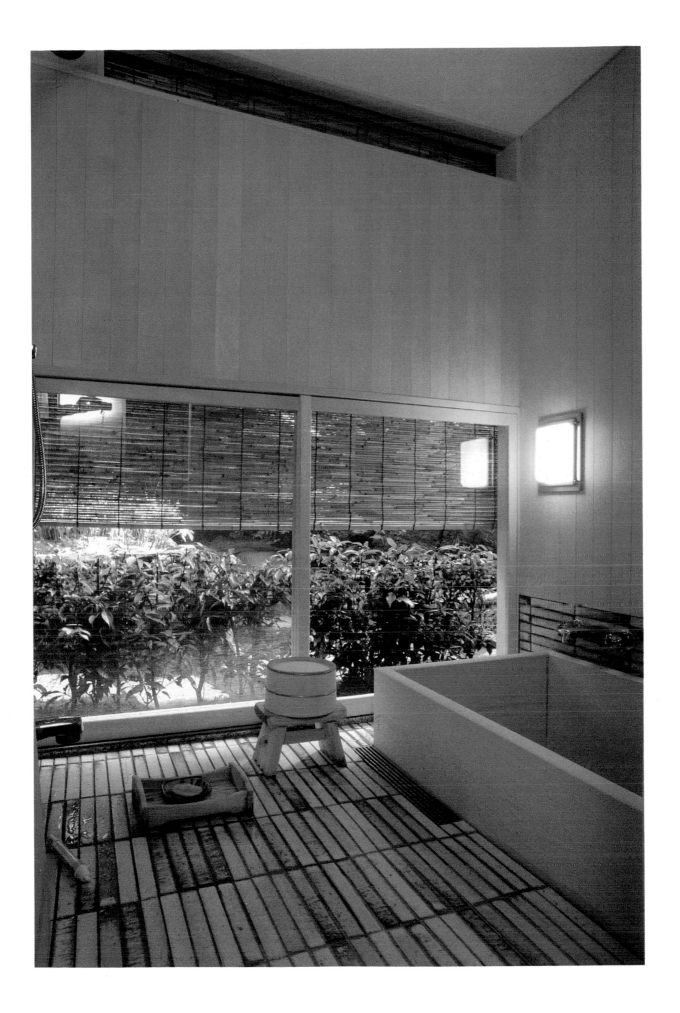

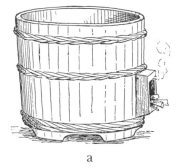

a

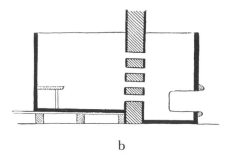

b

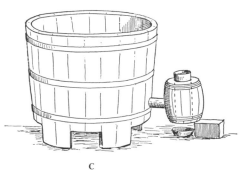

c

the hot chamber in which the fire is burning. In another form, a copper funnel or tube passes directly through the bottom of the bathing-tub (Fig. [a]). The bottom of this tube has a grating of wire; charcoal is then placed in the tube, and its combustion rapidly heats the water. A pan is placed below the tube to catch the coal and ashes that fall through. In a more elaborate form (Fig. [b]), the bath-tub is in two sections, separated by the partition of the room. These two sections are connected by a number of bamboo tubes or flues, so that the water may circulate freely. The section outside contains the fire-box, in which the fire is built; by this arrangement, the bather escapes the discomfort of the smoke from the fire.

A very excellent form of bathing-tub is shown in Fig. [c] in which outside the tub is a chamber not unlike a small wooden barrel closed at both ends; through this barrel runs a copper tube, in which a fire of charcoal is built. The barrel is connected with the bath-tub by a large bamboo tube, having a little square door within, which the bather may close if the water becomes too hot. In many cases a hood is arranged in such a way that the smoke from the fire is carried off. These tubs stand on a large wooden floor, the planks of which incline to a central gutter. Here the bather scrubs himself with a separate bucket of water, after having literally parboiled himself in water the temperature of which is so great that it is impossible for a foreigner to endure it.

A very common form of bath in the country consists of a large and shallow iron kettle, upon the top of which is secured a wooden extension, so as to give sufficient depth to the water within(Fig. [d]). The fire is built beneath the kettle,—the bather having a rack of wood which he sinks beneath him, and upon which he stands to protect his feet from burning. This tub is called a *Goyemon-buro,* named after Ishikawa Goyemon—a famous robber of Taiko's time, who was treated to a bath in boiling oil.

There are doubtless other forms of bath-tubs with conveniences for heating the water, but the forms here given comprise the principal kinds. There is no reason why similar conveniences might not be adopted in our country in cases where aqueducts or city supply is not available.

Although it was the standard a mere century ago, today the wooden tub is a highly prized luxury. Given the

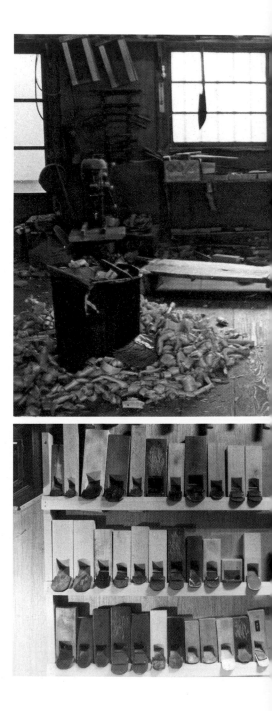

A fine wooden bathtub requires all the skill and artistry that Japanese carpenters lavish on building a teahouse or creating a work of art. *Below:* A free-standing tub of Japanese cypress, girded with copper bands, receives its finishing touches. *Left:* Sketches by Edward Sylvester Morse illustrate major types of Japanese bathtubs used in the late 1800s.

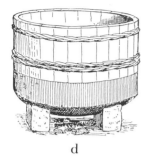

d

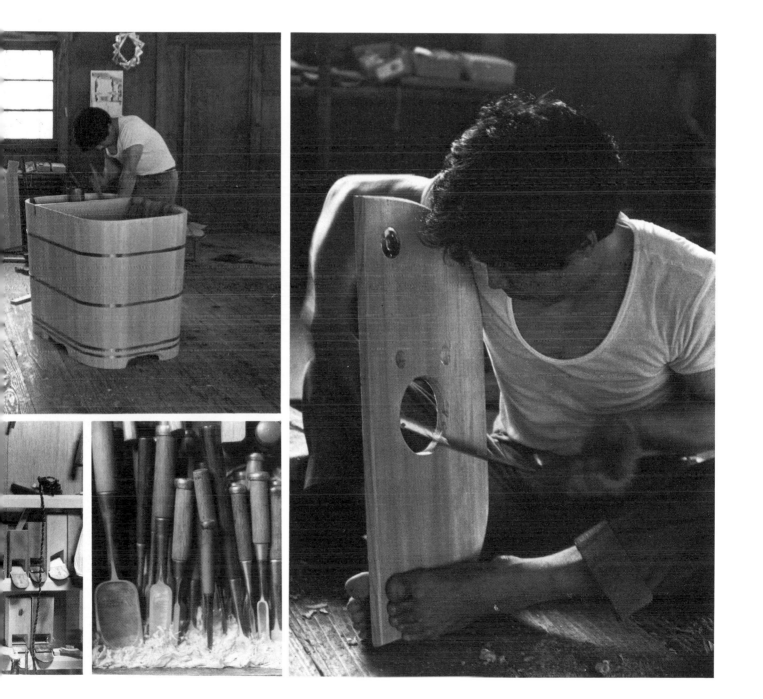

While the craftsmanship of fine carpenters is lavished on wooden tubs for expensive inns and wealthy homes, today most Japanese bathe at home in tubs made of steel or plastic.

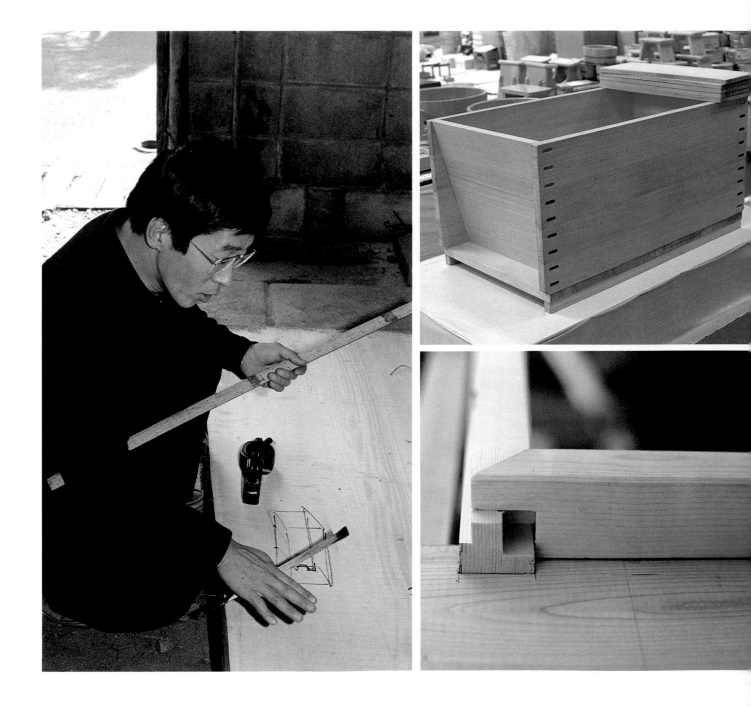

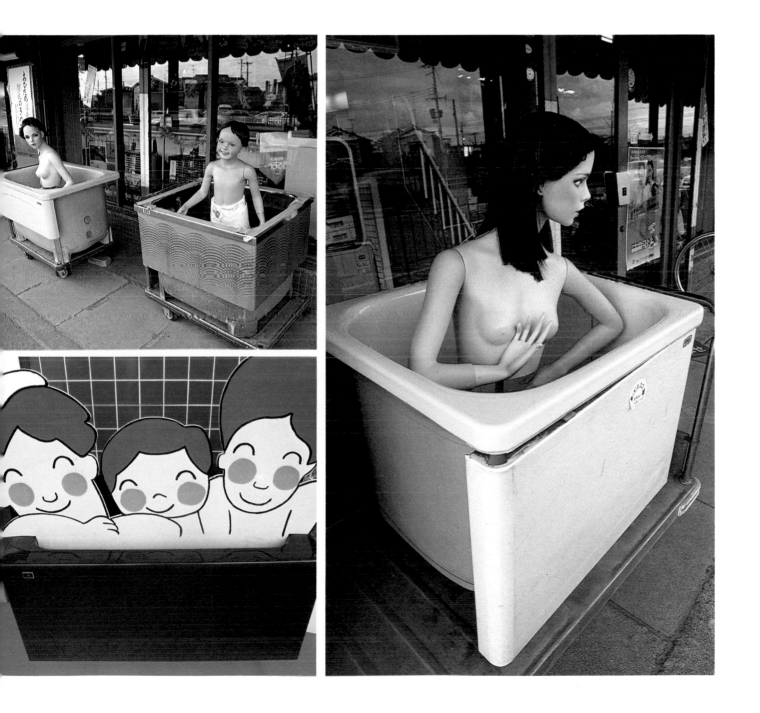

The domestic bath at its best: a tub of smooth, silken wood and a garden just outside the bathroom window. Even at home, where space is cramped, bathing is more fun when shared with another family member.

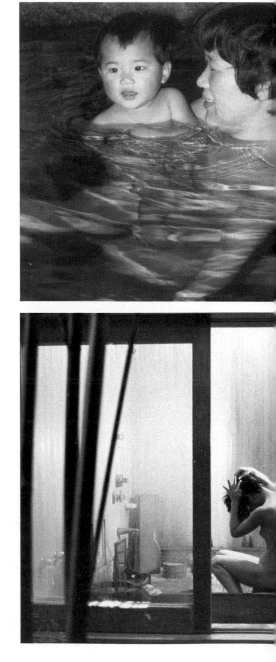

impracticality of wood—wooden tubs eventually disintegrate from long contact with water and must be replaced periodically—other materials gradually gained prominence after Japan was opened to the West in 1868. Nowadays, most tubs are manufactured of synthetic materials: tile, enamel, steel, and all manner of new plastic or fiberglass substances. Relatively inexpensive and easy to keep clean, the plastic tubs—generically called "poly-bath" (a shortening of "polyethylene bath")—have invaded virtually every Japanese home, where modern practicality has driven out traditional aesthetic considerations. On the other hand, the shower, perhaps the epitome of efficient bathing facilities, shows no signs of replacing the Japanese bath. While many home baths have shower heads, they are always installed in the washing area, not in the tub itself; showers seem destined to remain an accessory to the principal concern of every Japanese bather—a leisurely soak in deep hot water.

Modern methods of heating the bath water are almost as varied as the tubs themselves. Many domestic bathtubs are filled with hot water flowing from coil-type gas water-heaters, which do not store large quantities of hot water but rather heat it instantaneously on demand. More preferred, however, are built-in devices that heat and reheat the same water as it circulates in the tub. Cooler water flows from the bottom of the tub into the gas-fueled heating unit and emerges at a much higher temperature at the top of the tub. In this way, a tub may be filled initially with cold water, heated to the desired temperature, and reheated when it begins to cool. Also common are energy-conserving rooftop solar heaters that preheat the evening bath water on sunny days. In summer the water thus heated is hot enough to use as is; in winter it requires some reheating.

Although mass-produced plastic tubs have today, in accord with Gresham's Law of Coinage, driven out of common use the more costly other types of bathtub, still the fine wooden tub, painstakingly handcrafted of *hinoki* (Japanese cypress) or *maki* (Chinese black pine), remains the ideal. And since the ideal tub must not be placed in ill-suited surroundings, special care—not to mention expense—is necessary to provide the

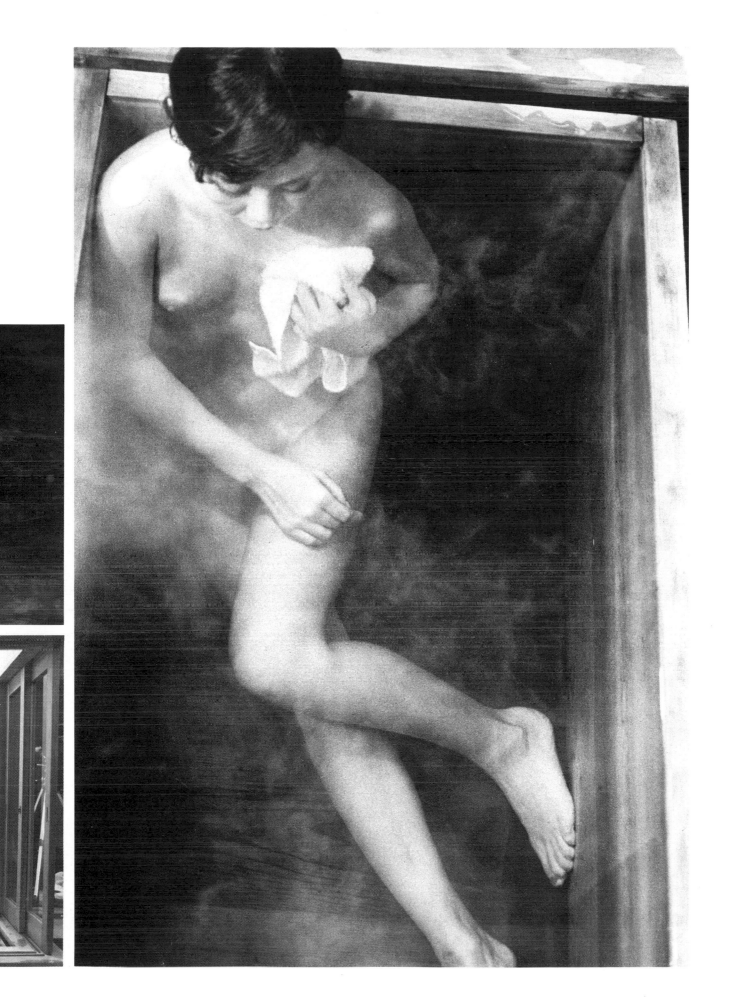

In "love hotels," (*below*) Japan's special contribution to sensuality and romance, baths enhance the atmosphere of eroticism with their sensuous shapes and luxurious settings and appointments.

Quietly, privately, a bather, (*right*) enjoys the clean, soothing refreshment of a bath at home. Except for the solitude, the pleasures are the same as at a public bath.

perfect environment for it. Few but the very wealthiest of families can afford the modernized version of the ideal traditional bathroom, for the single room alone may cost as much as sixty or seventy thousand dollars. The expense is not spent on the tub alone, of course, but on the design and execution of the entire space. Even the garden outside the bathroom window must be carefully cultivated to look its elegant best when viewed from the tub. Plumbing fixtures, tile work, floors of smooth handpicked stones, walls, illumination, small furnishings such as washbasins and low stools to sit on while washing outside the tub—all these features demand the same attention to design and craftsmanship as the tub itself.

Humbler folk may enjoy a whiff of the same luxury, however, by staying a night or two in one of Japan's finest *ryokan*, or inns, where every effort is made to insure the guest's comfort. But even luxury inns, able and willing to pay a premium price for bathrooms of exceptional elegance, often find it difficult to satisfy their needs. The managers of Kyoto's famed Tawaraya Inn, for example, gently complain that they must plan any bathroom renovation years in advance. Only one carpentry shop in Kyoto is able to build tubs and bathrooms that meet the Tawaraya's elevated standards and only a single craftsman can make the right type of wooden washbasin (and ever since he was declared a Living National Treasure he has been deluged with orders). Wood for the tub—rare *maki* or *hinoki*, and only that with the finest, straightest grain—must be ordered at least three or four years ahead so it can be properly aged before the carpentry begins. It comes as no surprise that the Tawaraya's program of refurbishing the bathrooms for its twenty or so guest rooms extends over a decade.

The result is well worth the wait. At an inn like the Tawaraya, every detail is in perfect harmony with the overall ambience of the whole bathroom, and the experience of a soak in one of the tubs there continues to evoke memories years later. The wood of the tub has been planed to the smoothness of silk, and when it is warmed by the hot water it softly envelops the human body like fine bedding. The moist cypress wood gives off

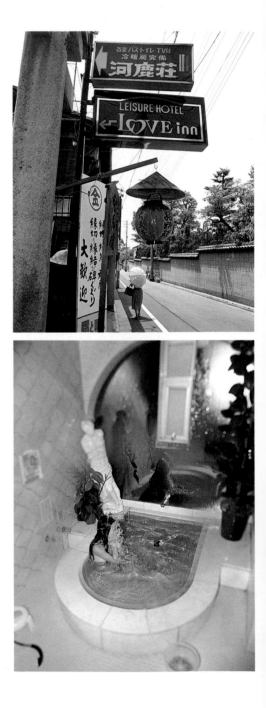

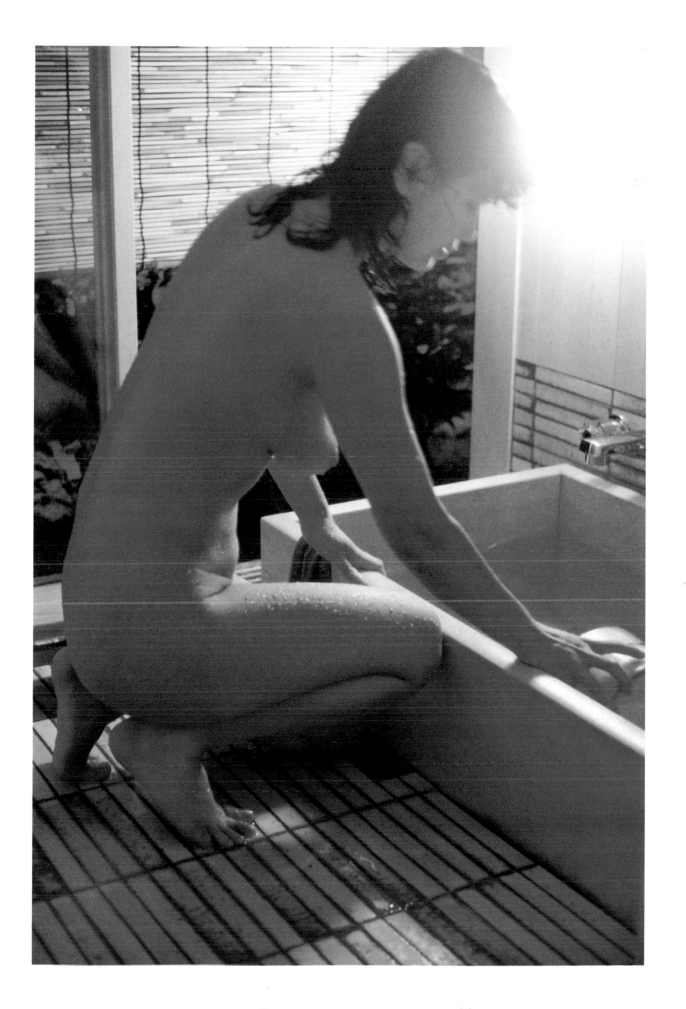

an indescribable natural perfume, a resinous aroma that never disappears, no matter how often the tub dries out. Rare is the foreign visitor, or the Japanese connoisseur of bathing experiences, who does not inquire of the innkeeper how and where he might find a similar tub to take home.

The rituals attending on domestic bathing in Japan are changing as rapidly as the wider society surrounding them. In earlier times, no one could bathe until the master of the house finished his bath. Rising from the first bath, when the water was hottest and cleanest, he would then be followed by a universally observed hierarchy of bathers: grandparents, eldest son, younger sons, daughters in order of declining age, and finally the wife of the house, followed at the very end by retainers and maids or other servants. Today, families are far less extended, and the hierarchy is broken down to fit better the realities of everyday life. Nowadays, in the typical small nuclear family, the mother of the house may often bathe first—late in the afternoon—so she can get her bath out of the way before setting about preparing dinner. Her children generally bathe next, and the father, who frequently does not return home until well after his wife and children have retired for the night, takes his bath last. If there are grandparents living with the family, the respect accorded their age generally allows them to bathe first.

So great is the Japanese love of bathing that a vast array of accessories has evolved to further enhance the experience at home. On the winter solstice, for example, citron—either the peel or the whole fruit—is added to the bath water in the belief that the citric acid and scented oil in the peel help heat the body and protect the skin from the approaching winter cold. On May 5, or Boys' Day, the fragrant leaves or roots of the sweet flag *(shobu)* are floated in the bath to help raise healthy boys capable of victory in contest *(shobu,* written with different ideograms, also means "victory"). This custom entered Japan from China, where the sweet flag was thought to have medicinal effects.

More recent innovations include bath salts that add color (generally emerald green or aqua) and scent (jasmine, floral mixes, and the like) and go by such brand names as Bath Clean. Or, one can save oneself a trip to a hot spring and have genuine *onsen* water trucked to the home bath. A less expensive alternative is to add several tablespoons of *yunohana* to your tub; this sometimes natural, usually manmade powder is supposed to transform your bath water into a silky smooth, sulphurous, mineral-laden "home *onsen.*" Perhaps the most creative innovation is the new sakè bath touted for its health benefits. More than two dozen brands of sakè are currently on sale for the express purpose of mixing into domestic baths.

Already it is not difficult to see the widening influence of Japanese bathing habits on American lives. California's hot-tub culture shows all the signs of enduring and outlasting its initial faddishness. American manufacturers have begun designing a far greater variety of tubs than ever before to replace the white porcelain oblong receptacle that was the standard item not long ago. Many of the new tubs are deeper, wider, and more comfortable. New types of water heaters provide hotter water in greater quantities with a lower expenditure of fuel, and experimentation is continuing with various built-in heating devices for reheating the water in hot tubs.

Gradually, Americans are inching closer and closer to adopting Japanese strategies for dealing with various aspects of daily life. We have quickly abandoned many of our earlier prejudices about Japanese people and their mores, replacing them with respect for the techniques the Japanese have developed for surmounting environmental and social pressures. We find ourselves turning increasingly toward Japan for inspiration and models for coping with contemporary problems and for addressing future needs. Having learned fuel economy from Japanese cars, management techniques from Japanese factories, and health enhancement from the Japanese diet, we are only now beginning to appreciate fully the physical and spiritual benefits of Japanese attitudes regarding cleanliness and bathing. Perhaps one of the most enduring blessings of our Eastward-looking education will be our immersion in the life-reinforcing hot water of the Japanese bath.

The following listing of Japanese hot springs, or *onsen*, is not intended to be comprehensive but to introduce more than a hundred of the most popular of the thousands of spas to be found in Japan. Beginning at the northernmost point of Hokkaido and extending in a generally southwesterly direction to southern Kyushu, this list includes most major *onsen* districts as well as many isolated hot springs that are renowned for some unusual geological or historical feature.

HOKKAIDO

WAKKANAI
The northernmost hot spring in Japan, located near Cape Noshappu.

MT. DAISETSU DISTRICT
On the slopes of Mt. Daisetsu in central Hokkaido are located the following *onsen:* Yukomanbetsu, Tenjinkyo, Aizankei, Sounkyo, Shirogane, Fukiage, and Tokachidake.

TOKACHIGAWA
A major resort center, located to the east of Obihiro City. Other nearby hot springs include Tsutsui, Chiyoda, and Makubetsu.

NOBORIBETSU
One of Hokkaido's largest and most popular *onsen* districts, comprising the hot-spring towns of Noboribetsu, Shin-noboribetsu, Karurusu, and the seaside resort of Shiraoirinkai.

NISEKO
A popular resort district in southeast Hokkaido that encompasses numerous hot-spring towns, including Kutchan, Hirafu, Niseko-goshiki, Yumoto, Konbu, Niseko-oyama, Konbugawa, Niseko-yunosato, and Niseko-yakushi.

YUNOKAWA
The principal hot-spring resort for residents of Hakodate City, located at the southernmost tip of Hokkaido.

AOMORI PREFECTURE

OSOREZAN
A hot spring located at the base of Mt. Osore, where for centuries superstitious Japanese have traveled to communicate with the spirits of dead relatives.

ASAMUSHI
One of the principal hot-spring resorts near Aomori City; the springs at Asamushi have been in constant use since the twelfth century.

HAKKODA DISTRICT
Mt. Hakkoda is one of the most popular resort areas of northern Honshu. Principal hot springs in the district include Tashirodai, Tashiro Motoyu, Hakkoda, Jogakura, Sugayu, Yachi, Sarukura, and the springs around the scenic Lake Towada.

HIROSAKI AND MT. IWAKI DISTRICT
The hot-spring towns surrounding Mt. Iwaki, near Hirosaki City, include Hyakusawa, Sanbon-yanagi, Hirosaki, Dake, and Yudan.

KUROISHI DISTRICT
The principal hot springs in the vicinity of Kuroishi City include Nuruyu, Ochiai, Itadome, Aoni, Nurukawa, and Choju.

IWATE PREFECTURE

HACHIMANTAI DISTRICT
The major hot springs on the Iwate side of the Hachiman Plateau in north-central Honshu include Gozaisho, Hachimantai, Matsukawa, Toshichi, and Iwatesan.

TSUNAGI
A popular resort near Morioka City, which traces its history to the twelfth-century military campaigns of Minamoto no Yoshiie.

HANAMAKI DISTRICT
A cluster of hot-spring towns around Hanamaki (itself one of the most popular *onsen* in the region), including Dai, Matsukura, Shidotaira, Osawa, Yamanokami, Takakurayama, Namari, and Shinnamari.

AKITA PREFECTURE

HACHIMANTAI DISTRICT
The boundary of Iwate and Akita prefectures crosses the highlands of the Hachiman Plateau. On the Akita side, the principal hot-spring resorts are Shibari, Zenikawa, Toroko, Akagawa, Sumikawa, Onuma, Goshogake, Obuka, Fukenoyu, and Tamagawa.

NYUTO DISTRICT
A popular cluster of hot-spring towns around Mt. Nyuto (also known as Mt. Eboshi), which includes Nyuto, Kuroyu, Taenoyu, Ogama, Ganiba, Magoroku, and Tsurunoyu.

OGA PENINSULA
The Oga Peninsula juts into the Japan Sea just north of Akita City; major seaside spas on the peninsula include Kamo, Kanegasaki, Toga, and Oga.

AKINOMIYA DISTRICT
Located in the mountains of southern Akita Prefecture, the Akinomiya district includes the hot-spring towns of Yunotai, Takanoyu, Inazumi, and Yunomata.

YAMAGATA PREFECTURE

AKAKURA
Frequented for skiing and other winter sports, as well as for its hot springs.

HIJIORI
Located northeast of the sacred mountain Gassan, Hijiori preserves the simple rustic atmosphere of its origins as a resting place for farmers and woodcutters.

YUNOHAMA
A popular seaside hot spring, the major resort for residents of nearby Tsuruoka City.

GINZAN
A small mountain resort located on the Ginzan River, in an area formerly known for its silver deposits.

TENDO
This town is known for the manufacture of *shogi* (Japanese chess) sets; a popular feature of the spas there is bathtubs shaped in the form of *shogi* pieces or pools in which the game is played on floating boards.

ZAO

One of Japan's most popular ski resorts, Zao is also famed for its hot springs, which are among the highest in altitude in northeastern Japan.

KAMINOYAMA

Originally the administrative seat of the local lord of the Matsudaira family, the *onsen* town of Kaminoyama still preserves much of its former historical atmosphere.

SHIRABU

Tracing its history back to the fourteenth century, the *onsen* town of Shirabu has long been one of the principal mountain resorts of the Yamagata region. Among the modern hotels lining its streets can still be found old thatched houses recalling its earlier history.

MIYAGI PREFECTURE

KURIKOMA DISTRICT

The principal hot-spring towns surrounding Mt. Kurikoma include Nuruyu, Yunokura, Yubama, and Komanoyu.

NARUGO DISTRICT

A thriving center of local handicrafts, Narugo is best known for its popular wooden *kokeshi* dolls, carried home as gifts by visitors to its many hot springs. The principal *onsen* towns in the area are Kawatabi, Higashi-narugo, Narugo, and Nakayamadaira.

ONIKUBI DISTRICT

Many of the springs in this area are known for their high temperatures and for their eruptions of powerful geysers and hot mud. Principal spas include Mitaki, Todoroki, Fukiage, and Miyazawa.

SAKUNAMI

For centuries, Sakunami has been a favorite spa for residents of nearby Sendai City. The resort is known for its large open-air rock grotto baths along the Hirose River.

FUKUSHIMA PREFECTURE

IIZAKA

One of the largest and most popular *onsen* towns in the Tohoku region of northern Japan. More than 120 hotels cluster along the Surigami River, which flows through the center of the town.

AZUMA DISTRICT

Located slightly southwest of Fukushima City, the Azuma district contains one of the most abundant concentrations of hot springs in central Japan. The principal *onsen* towns are Takayu, Tsuchiyu, Fudoyu, Yokomuki, Nakanosawa, Numajiri, and Dake.

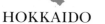

179

HOKKAIDO

HONSHU

KYUSHU

SHIKOKU

J A P A N

BANDAI PLATEAU AND LAKE INAWASHIRO

The district north and west of Lake Inawashiro contains some of the most popular resorts of the area, including Kawakami, Kita-shiobara, Higashiyama, Ashinomaki, and Yunogami.

TOCHIGI PREFECTURE

NASU DISTRICT

Drawn by the beautiful scenery, cool air, and year-round recreational facilities, many wealthy Japanese—including the imperial family—have built villas in the Nasu mountains. Among the hot-spring resorts in this volcanic range are Nasu Yumoto, Takao, Yawata, Asahi, Kita, Benten, Omaru, Sandogoya, and Itamuro.

SHIOBARA DISTRICT
This well-known cluster of hot-spring towns along the Hoki River includes Kami-shiobara, Naka-shiobara, Furumachi, Monzen, Hataori, Shionoyu, Shiogama, and Fukuwata.

KINUGAWA
One of the most popular hot-spring resorts in the area immediately north of Tokyo, Kinugawa has more than fifty hotels, many of them high-rise structures built along both banks of the narrow Kinu River.

CHUZENJI
Along the shores of beautiful Lake Chuzenji, located just above the town of Nikko, are more than fifteen hot-spring inns and hotels. This is a popular overnight stop for tourists visiting the shrines and historical sites of Nikko.

NIKKO YUMOTO
Another popular hot-spring resort for visitors to Nikko is Nikko Yumoto. Its springs have been known for more than twelve centuries; in recent years, the district has also attracted skiers, hikers, and campers.

GUMMA PREFECTURE

IKAHO
Built along the steep rocky slopes of Mt. Haruna, Ikaho is a conveniently located retreat for Tokyo residents. The spa is known for its beautiful scenery and for its large outdoor baths.

MIKUNI DISTRICT
The Mikuni Pass divides the three prefectures of Gumma, Niigata, and Nagano. Among the principal hot-spring resorts on the Gumma side are Yujuku, Akaiwa, Sarugakyo, Kawafuru, and Hoshi.

MINAKAMI DISTRICT
Minakami is a flourishing resort town of more than thirty hotels and many smaller inns. Popular nearby hot-spring resorts include Yunoko-ya, Tanigawa, and Yubiso.

TAKARAGAWA
Located only a couple of miles from Minakami, Takaragawa boasts one of Japan's largest and most beautiful *rotenburo,* or open-air baths. It is spectacular in the autumn and the winter when one can sit in the hot waters as snow falls.

SHIMA
Along with Ikaho and Kusatsu, Shima has long been one of the most celebrated spas in the region immediately north of Tokyo. It is particularly popular in spring and autumn, when bathers enjoy the colorful scenery from large outdoor hot-spring pools.

KUSATSU
Among the nearly two hundred hostelries in Kusatsu are fine luxury hotels and small old-fashioned inns. Popular as a resort since the twelfth century, Kusatsu's extremely hot natural springs are said to be effective in curing any human affliction—except love.

MANZA
Situated more than 5,500 feet above sea level and surrounded by steep mountains, Manza is popular both for its ski slopes and for its hot natural springs.

TOKYO
Within the city of Tokyo are twenty-six springs, which in most cases provide bathers with natural hot water. Among the most accessible bathhouses are the Azabu Juban Onsen (in Azabu), Kannon Onsen (Asakusa), Juniso Tennen Onsen (Shinjuku), Ebisu-yu (Shibuya), and Ikegami Onsen (Nishi-kamata).

KANAGAWA PREFECTURE

HAKONE DISTRICT
Hakone, in the eastern foothills of Mt. Fuji, has long been one of the resort areas most popular with Tokyo residents; it is well known for its scenic beauty and fine accommodations. Among its noted hot-spring towns are Hakone Yumoto, Tonosawa, Ohiradai, Miyanoshita, Gora, Kowakidani, Ashinoko, and Sengokubara.

YUGAWARA
Located along the coast near Atami and extending into the hills toward Hakone, Yugawara is a hot-spring resort of great scenic beauty and tranquility. Barely more than an hour by train from Tokyo, the town boasts more than 130 hostelries, including several of Japan's most elegant inns.

SHIZUOKA PREFECTURE

ATAMI
One of Japan's largest hot-springs resorts, Atami boasts nearly four hundred hotels and inns of all sizes, with accommodations for virtually every taste and budget. Natural hot water flows to the hotels from more than three hundred different springs. Atami's easy accessibility from Tokyo makes it a popular spot for overnight trips and festive weekends. Crowded year-round, Atami's atmosphere tends to be boisterous and raucous in its central district; on the outskirts of town and in the hills above it are inns and villas of great elegance, sited in peaceful spots overlooking the sea.

ITO
Only slightly smaller than Atami, Ito is no less popular as a holiday resort among Tokyo residents. Its hotels built up the steep slopes command wonderful views of Sagami Bay and the surrounding mountains.

IZU PENINSULA
The Izu Peninsula contains scores of hot-spring resorts of all sizes. Many seaside towns along the eastern coast offer fine beaches as well as excellent spas; among the most popular are Okawa, Hokkawa, Atagawa, Katase, Inatori, and Imaihama.

SHIMODA
Located at the southern tip of the Izu Peninsula is the resort of Shimoda, where Tokyo residents delight in the semitropical climate and fine luxury hotels. An important port in the nineteenth century, Shimoda was the site of Townsend Harris's first U.S. consulate in Japan.

CENTRAL IZU
The mountainous spine of the Izu Peninsula is dotted with many hot-spring towns and resorts where wealthy Tokyoites have established vil-

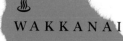

las and varied recreational facilities, including fine golf courses. The principal spas, many of which figure in Yasunari Kawabata's famous novel *The Izu Dancer*, include Izu-nagaoka, Ohito, Shuzenji, Shiroiwa, and Yugashima.

NIIGATA PREFECTURE

SENAMI
A popular hot-spring resort on the Japan Sea. The town faces a broad sandy beach that is broken only by strands of pine trees and that is crowded with swimmers every summer.

MT. YAHIKO
Mt. Yahiko rises abruptly along the coast of the Japan Sea south of Niigata City. The hot spring is on the inland slope of the mountain, facing away from the sea. A ropeway links the town to the top of the mountain, which commands an impressive view of the sea and Sado Island floating in the distance.

ECHIGO YUZAWA
Located on the Niigata side of Mikuni Pass, Echigo Yuzawa is famed as the locale of Yasunari Kawabata's novel *Snow Country*. Aside from the geographical setting, however, little remains of the rustic hot-spring town described in the novel. Today, Echigo Yuzawa is a stop on the "bullet train," is bisected by broad highways, and is full of large high-rise hotels.

MYOKO PLATEAU
Mt. Myoko, at 8,025 feet, is one of the highest peaks in Niigata. Its slopes and surrounding mountains offer some of Japan's finest skiing and are dotted with hot-spring resorts as well. The principal springs in the area are Myoko, Ikenotaira, Akakura, Seki, and Tsubame.

HAKUBA
A popular ski resort, known also for its large *rotenburo*, or open-air hot-spring bath. Beyond Hakuba, deeper in the mountains, is Renge Onsen, also famous for its great *rotenburo* and scenic hiking trails.

YAMANASHI PREFECTURE

FUEFUKI DISTRICT
Named for the Fuefuki River, which cuts through the mountains northwest of Mt. Fuji, the area is full of well-known spas. Among the most popular of them are Kasugai, Isawa, Kawaura, Mitomi, and Amashina.

SHIMOBE
Shimobe is famous in Japanese history as one of the "hidden springs" where the sixteenth-century warlord Takeda Shingen rested his armies between battles. Then, as now, the waters of Shimobe were thought to be particularly efficacious in healing wounds.

NAGANO PREFECTURE

TATESHINA DISTRICT
The high plateau south of Mt. Tateshina and northwest of Mt. Yatsu in the Japan Alps is the site of one of the richest concentrations of hot springs in Japan. The springs are popular with hikers and campers in summer and with skiers in winter. Principal spas in the area include Tateshina, Takinoyu, Shinyu, Yokoya, Meiji, Shibukawa, Shibu, and Shibunoyu.

LAKE SUWA DISTRICT
On the shores of Lake Suwa, with its historic shrine, are the two large hot-spring resorts of Kami-suwa and Shimo-suwa.

MARUKO DISTRICT
In the mountains along the Chikuma River near Ueda in northern Nagano Prefecture lie a number of hot springs that have been used for centuries. The principal spas in the area are Reisenji, Oshio, Kakeyu, Bessho, Kutsukake, and Tazawa.

YUDANAKA AND SHIBU DISTRICT
The Joshinetsu-kogen National Park in the northernmost area of Nagano Prefecture teems with hot-spring resorts that are well equipped with facilities for skiing and other winter and summer sports. Major springs in the area are Yudanaka, Hoshikawa, Andai, Shibu, Honami, Kanbayashi, and Jigokudani.

ASAMA AND UTSUKUSHIGAHARA DISTRICT
Two popular hot-spring resorts in the vicinity of Matsumoto City are Asama and Utsukushi-gahara. Asama is in the northern suburbs of the city and Utsukushigahara is located on a high plateau above it, affording magnificent views of the Northern Japan Alps.

KAMIKOCHI AND NORIKURA PLATEAU
Beautiful scenery and excellent resort facilities make Kamikochi and the surrounding Norikura Plateau one of Japan's most popular alpine retreats. Major springs in the area include Norikura, Shirahone, and Kamikochi.

AICHI PREFECTURE

YUYA
A small hot-spring resort in the mountains east of Nagoya. Nearby is the Horai-ji temple, an eighth-century edifice of the Shingon sect, and the scenic Horai Gorge.

KIRA
A seaside *onsen* resort on Mikawa Bay, southeast of Nagoya.

SHINOSHIMA
A hot-spring resort on a tiny island in Mikawa Bay, located just off the southernmost tip of the Chita Peninsula. In addition to the spa, the island is noted for its fine beaches and small fishing villages.

TOYAMA PREFECTURE

OGAWA MOTOYU
An old but hard-to-reach spa high in the mountains above the town of Tomari on the Hokuriku Railway Line that follows the northern coast of Honshu along the Japan Sea. The hot spring and its large open-air bathing pool are particularly popular with hikers and mountaineers.

KUROBE-UNAZUKI DISTRICT
Many small hot springs are to be found along the Kurobe River, which flows into the Japan

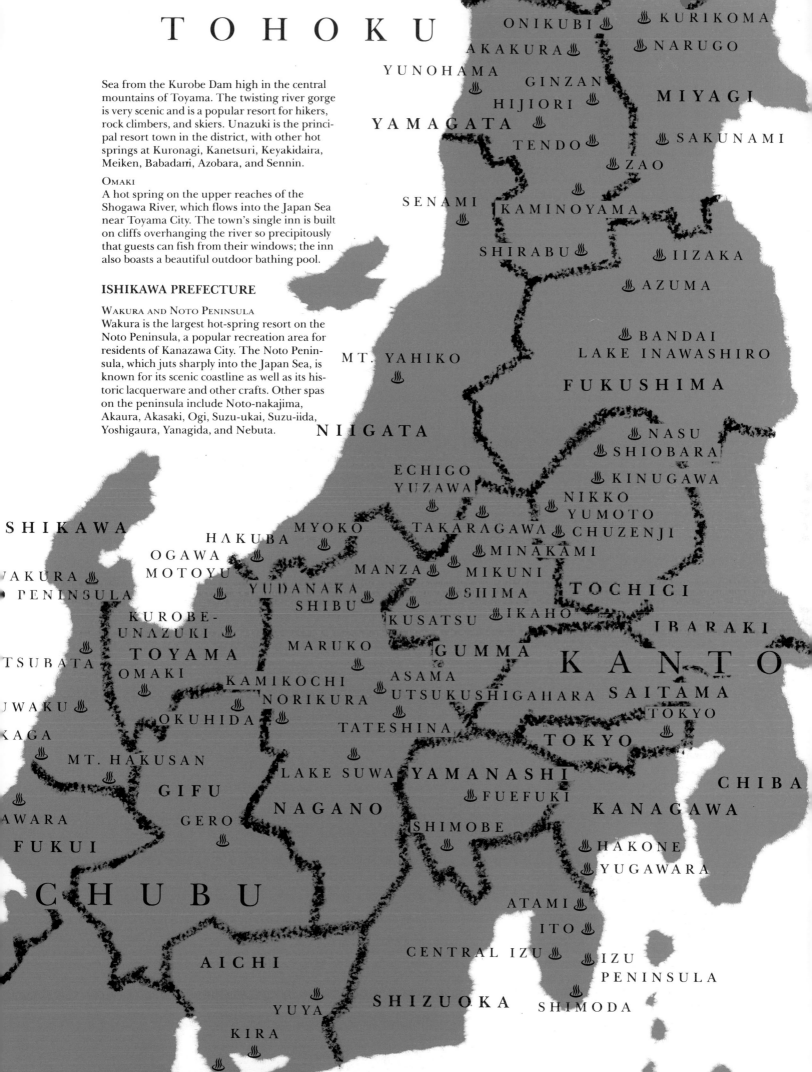

T O H O K U

Sea from the Kurobe Dam high in the central mountains of Toyama. The twisting river gorge is very scenic and is a popular resort for hikers, rock climbers, and skiers. Unazuki is the principal resort town in the district, with other hot springs at Kuronagi, Kanetsuri, Keyakidaira, Meiken, Babadarri, Azobara, and Sennin.

OMAKI
A hot spring on the upper reaches of the Shogawa River, which flows into the Japan Sea near Toyama City. The town's single inn is built on cliffs overhanging the river so precipitously that guests can fish from their windows; the inn also boasts a beautiful outdoor bathing pool.

ISHIKAWA PREFECTURE

WAKURA AND NOTO PENINSULA
Wakura is the largest hot-spring resort on the Noto Peninsula, a popular recreation area for residents of Kanazawa City. The Noto Peninsula, which juts sharply into the Japan Sea, is known for its scenic coastline as well as its historic lacquerware and other crafts. Other spas on the peninsula include Noto-nakajima, Akaura, Akasaki, Ogi, Suzu-ukai, Suzu-iida, Yoshigaura, Yanagida, and Nebuta.

ONIKUBI · KURIKOMA
AKAKURA · NARUGO
YUNOHAMA · GINZAN · MIYAGI
HIJIORI
YAMAGATA · TENDO · SAKUNAMI
ZAO
SENAMI · KAMINOYAMA
SHIRABU · IIZAKA
AZUMA
MT. YAHIKO · BANDAI
LAKE INAWASHIRO
FUKUSHIMA
NIIGATA · NASU
SHIOBARA
ECHIGO · KINUGAWA
YUZAWA · NIKKO
YUMOTO
MYOKO · TAKARAGAWA · CHUZENJI
HAKUBA · MINAKAMI
OGAWA
MOTOYU · MANZA · MIKUNI
SHIKAWA · YUDANAKA · SHIMA · TOCHIGI
SHIBU · KUSATSU · IKAHO · IBARAKI
WAKURA · KUROBE-
PENINSULA · UNAZUKI · MARUKO · GUMMA · KANTO
TSUBATA · TOYAMA · ASAMA · SAITAMA
OMAKI · KAMIKOCHI · UTSUKUSHIGAHARA · TOKYO
UWAKU · NORIKURA · TOKYO
KAGA · OKUHIDA · TATESHINA · TOKYO
MT. HAKUSAN · LAKE SUWA · YAMANASHI · CHIBA
GIFU · FUEFUKI · KANAGAWA
AWARA · NAGANO · SHIMOBE
GERO · HAKONE
FUKUI · YUGAWARA
ATAMI
ITO
CHUBU · CENTRAL IZU · IZU
PENINSULA
AICHI
YUYA · SHIZUOKA · SHIMODA
KIRA
SHINOSHIMA

Tsubata District

Located a mile or so northeast of Kanazawa City is a cluster of *onsen* towns, including Tsubata, Asada, Kurami, Kurikara, Morimoto, Aoi, and Yakushigaoka.

Yuwaku

A hot-spring town located on a plateau southeast of Kanazawa and popular with residents of that city. In addition to its modern hotels, the town has preserved a number of centuries-old hostelries. A nearby attraction is Edo Village, a collection of well-restored farmhouses and other architecturally significant buildings from the Edo period (1603–1868).

Mt. Hakusan District

The mountains of central Ishikawa Prefecture are famous for their dense forests, scenic river gorges, and challenging hiking or rock-climbing trails. Mt. Hakusan, one of the mountains sacred to the esoteric sects of Shingon Buddhism, comprises five peaks: Gozenmine (8,865 feet), Onanjimine (8,681 feet), Tsurugigamine (8,714 feet), Bessan (7,870 feet), and Sannomine (6,437 feet). The principal hot springs in the area are Hakusan-ichirino, Shin-iwama, Chugu, Shiramine, and Hakusan.

Kaga District

The central plain between Kanazawa and Fukui cities was historically one of Japan's most fertile and most productive regions, supporting the economic power of the Maeda family, which ruled the district from Kanazawa. The area abounds in historical sites and crafts villages. Among the principal hot springs are Awazu, Katayamazu, Yamashiro, Yamanaka, and Kagamitani.

FUKUI PREFECTURE

Awara

Located slightly to the north of Fukui City, the Awara spa is the principal resort for residents of Fukui. Its more than seventy-five hotels also draw their clientele from Kanazawa, Kyoto, and Osaka. Other smaller spas in the area include Yoshizaki and Tojinbo.

GIFU PREFECTURE

Okuhida District

Okuhida, in the northeast corner of Gifu Prefecture, contains several of the highest peaks of Japan's Northern Alps. The spas in the district are some of the highest in altitude, and are frequented by hikers and campers in summer and by skiers in winter. Principal *onsen* include Hirayu, Shin-hirayu, Fukuji, Tochio, and Shin-hodaka.

Gero

Located on the Hida River, formerly serving as a major post-town on the old mountain road connecting the cities of Nagoya and Takayama, Gero is today a flourishing resort town. Its springs, with their ancient history of healing powers, have attracted farmers and mountain villagers for centuries. Today, tourists come to Gero to relax in its spas, enjoy the beautiful surrounding scenery, and examine the well-preserved historical farmhouses of the region.

MIE PREFECTURE

Nagashima

Nagashima, slightly southeast of Nagoya, is one of the principal *onsen* resorts for residents of that city. Among its main attractions are a hot-spring pool large enough to accommodate two thousand bathers at one time.

Yunoyama

An ancient hot spring, known historically as Shikanoyu, used by residents of the Yamato Plain more than twelve hundred years ago. Visitors from Kyoto, Osaka, Nara, and Nagoya are still drawn to its waters and lovely scenery.

SHIGA PREFECTURE

Lake Biwa District

The hot-spring towns along the southern shores of Lake Biwa—Biwako, Imahama, Ogoto, and Shirataki—were favorite retreats for residents of the ancient capital of Kyoto. Today, they are still popular resorts, widely known for their bowling alleys, gambling casinos, Turkish baths, and other recreational facilities.

KYOTO PREFECTURE

Yunohana

Located near Kameoka, a short train ride from Kyoto, Yunohana is a popular spot for daylong outings. In earlier times, it served as a cool country retreat from the stifling summer heat of Kyoto.

Kizu

Kizu is located on the Tango Peninsula, which extends into the Japan Sea. Its spas and sandy beaches make it a pleasant resort, especially in summertime.

NARA PREFECTURE

Yoshino

The lovely hills and valleys of the Yoshino district have inspired some of Japan's most beloved classical poetry and dramatic literature. In springtime, the entire region bursts into magnificent color with its cherry blossoms, and the autumn scenery is no less spectacular. The region is rich with historical sites, including hundreds of temples, shrines, and palaces, in addition to numerous fine hot springs.

Tosenji

Located on the Totsugawa River, which winds its way through the mountains of Nara and Wakayama prefectures, Tosenji was an ancient retreat for aristocrats and religious recluses from the cities of Kyoto and Nara. The area is still known for its tranquility and beautiful scenery.

NAGATO

YAMAGUCHI

KAWATANA

WAKAYAMA PREFECTURE

ARITA

A popular *onsen* on the western coast of the Kii Peninsula that is a favorite resort of fishermen drawn there by rich fishing grounds. A distinctive feature of Arita is its gondola baths—tub-lined gondolas suspended from a ropeway that provide a breathtaking view of the coastal cliffs.

YUNOMINE AND KAWAYU

Both of these inland *onsen* resorts are located near the scenic gorge of the Totsugawa River, which cuts through the central mountains of the Kii Peninsula. Rich in historical and religious sites, including the shrines of Kumano Hongu, the area was for centuries a favorite retreat of aristocrats of the Nara and Kyoto courts.

SHIRAHAMA

One of Japan's best-known seaside *onsen* resorts, Shirahama ranks with Atami and Beppu in variety of hostelries and recreational facilities. Shirahama's warm climate and excellent fishing draw visitors year-round to its sandy beaches and fine hot-spring hotels.

KATSUURA

Scenic Kumano Bay, dotted with small islands, and the hot-srping towns along its coastline make this area of southern Kii Peninsula a popular resort. The principal *onsen* towns are Taiji, Natsuyama, Yukawa, and Katsuura, where a major attraction is the cave baths along the rocky coast.

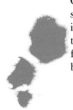

KINOSAKI
KIZU
LAKE BIWA
IWAI
NAGASHIMA
YUMURA
KYOTO
SHIGA
MISASA
YUNOHANA
YUNOYAMA
MATSUE
TOTTORI
KAIKE
HYOGO
MIE
TAMATSUKURI
OKUTSU
TAKARAZUKA
TAISHA
YUBARA
ARIMA
KINKI
SHIMANE
OKAYAMA
OSAKA
YOSHINO
CHUGOKU
NARA
ARITA
TOSENJI
HIROSHIMA
KAGAWA
WAKAYAMA
YUKI
SHIONOE
YUMOTO
KAWAYU
YUNOMINE
TOKUSHIMA
SHIRAHAMA   KATSUURA
EHIME
DOGO
KOCHI
OKUDOGO
KOCHI

SHIKOKU

HYOGO PREFECTURE

ARIMA

Located on the northern slopes of Mt. Rokko above Kobe, Arima is one of Japan's oldest spas, with references to it in many ancient historical records. The springs were favored by aristocrats of the Nara and Kyoto courts for their medicinal properties and for their peaceful environs.

TAKARAZUKA

Located between Osaka and Kobe, Takarazuka serves as a convenient retreat for residents of both cities. Its parks are a favorite site for family outings, and its fine hotels make it a popular destination of newlyweds. Takarazuka is also the home of the famed Takarazuka all-female opera and dance revue.

KINOSAKI

Kinosaki has for centuries been one of the most popular resorts on the Japan Sea coast, favored particularly by poets and writers for its quiet setting and for the variety of bathing experiences available at its seven different springs.

YUMURA

Along with Kinosaki, Yumura is one of the best-known *onsen* resorts along the coast of the Japan Sea. The town boasts a variety of different springs, which are said to be particularly effective in treating rheumatism and gastro-intestinal diseases.

TOTTORI PREFECTURE

IWAI

Slightly to the west of Yumura is Iwai, where the springs have been in use for over a thousand years. The nearby shore of the Japan Sea is noted for its sandy beaches and great dunes.

MISASA

Together with Kinosaki and Yumura, Misasa is one of the most renowned hot-spring resorts along the Japan Sea. Its many inns and hotels are popular with families, honeymooners, and other holiday travelers.

KAIKE

Located along a sandy strand fronting on the Japan Sea near Yonago, Kaike is as popular for its beaches as for its hot springs. The view of Mt. Oyama across the bay is particularly lovely from this spot.

OKAYAMA PREFECTURE

OKUTSU

Okutsu is situated in the central mountains that bisect western Honshu, separating the fertile plains along the Japan Sea to the north from the plains along the Inland Sea to the south. It is a popular resort for residents of Himeji, Okayama, Fukuyama, and other port cities of the Inland Sea. The Takeda River flows through the town, and large open-air hot-spring pools have been built along its banks.

YUBARA DISTRICT

A popular cluster of *onsen* towns is to be found around Yubara in the mountains of central Okayama. This area is near the watershed of central Honshu, with some rivers flowing down to the Inland Sea and others flowing north toward the Japan Sea. The principal spas in the region are Maga, Taru, Goroku, and Yubara.

SHIMANE PREFECTURE

MATSUE

Matsue is the lovely provincial city where American writer Lafcadio Hearn made his home after adopting Japanese citizenship and the pen name Koizumi Yakumo. His home, located near the moat surrounding Matsue Castle, is still preserved there.

TAMATSUKURI

This well-known *onsen* resort along the Japan Sea coast is a short train ride from the city of Matsue. The history of the Tamatsukuri spa extends back at least thirteen hundred years; today it is a bustling resort town, full of well-equipped inns, restaurants, and recreational facilities.

TAISHA

A relatively small hot-spring town, but a popular one because of its proximity to the ancient Great Shrines of Izumo. Other nearby *onsen* include Koryo, Tachikuekyo, Hanakura, and Oda.

HIROSHIMA PREFECTURE

YUKI

An inland resort town frequented by the citizens of Hiroshima City. The hot springs at Yuki are believed to have been in continuous use since the beginning of the ninth century.

YAMAGUCHI PREFECTURE

NAGATO DISTRICT

One of the most scenic stretches of the Japan Sea coastline is near the port town of Nagato in western Yamaguchi Prefecture, where rocky peninsulas jut into the island-studded sea. The district is also noted for its fine ceramics, particularly those produced in the town of Hagi. Principal hot-spring resorts in the district include Nagato Yumoto, Tawarayama, Ofuku, Omishima, Kiwado, and Yuyawan.

KAWATANA

Located near the western tip of Honshu, Kawatana is one of the most popular *onsen* in the area between Nagato and Shimonoseki. The fine sandy beaches near the town also draw visitors from Hiroshima and northern Kyushu.

KAGAWA PREFECTURE

SHIONOE YUMOTO

Unlike the area of central Honshu facing it across the Inland Sea, the island of Shikoku is not richly endowed with hot springs. One of Shikoku's best-known springs is Shionoe Yumoto, located in the mountains of Kagawa Prefecture near the border with Tokushima. The area is noted for its scenery and the fine fishing in the mountain streams.

KOCHI PREFECTURE

KOCHI

In the environs of Kochi City, on the southern

coast of Shikoku, are a number of *onsen* towns popular with local residents. Chief among them are Inosawa, Senmai, Yumeno, Wakamiya, and Engyoji. The district is also popular with vacationers for its sandy beaches and semitropical climate.

EHIME PREFECTURE

Dogo and Okudogo

Located within the city limits of Matsuyama, the Dogo spa is one of the oldest and most celebrated in the region. It was known as a distant resort by aristocrats of the Kyoto court and during the late nineteenth century attained instant fame as the setting of Natsume Soseki's popular novel *Botchan*. Okudogo, located in the mountains a couple of miles west of Matsuyama City, is a newer resort, with large hotels famed for their enormous "jungle baths."

FUKUOKA PREFECTURE

Futsukaichi

Located just to the south of Fukuoka City, near the ancient shrine of Dazaifu, the *onsen* at Futsukaichi (formerly known as Suita) is one of the oldest in the country. Poems referring to it appear in the eighth-century imperial anthology *Manyoshu*, and the spa has always been a popular stopover for pilgrims to Dazaifu.

Harazuru

A cluster of popular hot springs in the central region of northern Kyushu has Harazuru at its center; other nearby spas include Yoshii, Chikugogawa, and Chikuzen-hayashida.

SAGA PREFECTURE

Takeo

Takeo boasts an ancient heritage: legend has it that the prehistoric empress Jingo bathed there before launching her invasion of Korea. In premodern times, Takeo was also known as Tsukasaki, and was referred to as such by Engelbert Kaempfer in his seventeenth-century journals.

Ureshino

References to this popular spring are to be found in Japan's earliest historical records. The town today is a flourishing resort, boasting more than eighty hotels and inns, some with great open-air bathing pools.

NAGASAKI PREFECTURE

Unzen

One of the best-known hot-spring resorts in Japan. Unzen's fame has been spread abroad by the many foreign visitors to its fine hotels, golf courses, and scenic attractions. One of the earliest Europeans to write about Unzen was Engelbert Kaempfer, who visited the springs during his sojourn in Nagasaki in 1691–92. Located on a mountainous peninsula east of Nagasaki, Unzen has a multitude of springs of differing chemical properties. The oldest of these have been in continuous use for more than twelve hundred years.

FUKUOKA

FUTSUKAICHI

OITA

BEPPU

YUFUIN

HARAZURU

SAGA

TAKEO

KUJU

MT. ASO

URESHINO

MT. ASO

YAMAGA

NAGASAKI

SHIMABARA

UNZEN

KUMAMOTO

OBAMA

MIYAZAKI

HINAGU

EBINO

MT. KIRISHIMA

SHINKAWA

KAGOSHIMA

IBUSUKI

KYUSHU

OBAMA

Obama is a resort on the western coast of the Unzen Peninsula. While visitors flock to its spas year-round, its sandy beaches make it especially popular during the summer months.

SHIMABARA

Located on the eastern shore of the Unzen Peninsula, Shimabara is celebrated for its beautiful seacoast and its handsome castle. During the early seventeenth century, Shimabara was an important center of Christian missionary activity and was the site of the Tokugawa government. Today, it is a small but flourishing port town, from which ferries service the many tiny islands of the Ariake Sea.

OITA PREFECTURE

BEPPU DISTRICT

Beppu is rivaled only by Atami as one of the largest hot-spring resorts in Japan. Located on the eastern coast of Kyushu, it is an important port for boats traversing the Inland Sea, and together with the adjacent towns Beppu boasts nearly one thousand hotels, inns, and other hostelries. Nearly every variety of geothermal spring is to be found in the vicinity of Beppu, and some of the springs are the hottest in Japan; the area is known for its great geothermal "hells," hot-mud springs, geysers, and springs along the sandy beaches. The many "hells"—sites where steam and hot water burst out of the ground—are great tourist attractions, as are the great open-air bathing pools and "jungle baths" constructed in huge indoor enclosures that resemble greenhouses. Other resort towns in the immediate vicinity include Kankaiji, Horita, Hamawaki, Kannawa, Myoban, Shibaseki, and Kamegawa.

YUFUIN

Located on a plateau on the other side of Mt. Yufu from Beppu, the resort of Yufuin is far smaller and quieter than the rather raucous Beppu. It has experienced considerable development in recent years, and now has more than forty hotels. many of which have lovely wings in traditional Japanese style.

KUJU DISTRICT AND MT. ASO

Mt. Aso is a huge volcanic crater occupying the central highlands of Kyushu. Its plateaus and foothills spill into Oita, Kumamoto, and Miyazaki prefectures, and the entire region is richly endowed with geothermal springs. The eastern slopes of Mt. Aso, in Oita Prefecture, are known as the Kuju Highlands and are covered with broad open expanses of grasslands, golf courses, livestock ranches, and campgrounds. Some of the principal hot-spring resorts in the area are Chojabaru, Kannojigoku, Makinoto, Hossho, Hokke-in, Nagayu, Kuju-akagawa, and Hizenyu.

KUMAMOTO PREFECTURE

MT. ASO DISTRICT

The western slopes of Mt. Aso on the Kumamoto side are no less rich in *onsen* than those on the Oita side. Some of the principal springs are Toshita, Aso-uchinomaki, Aso-akamizu, Tochino-ki, Yunotani, Tarutama, and Jigoku.

YAMAGA DISTRICT

Further west of Mt. Aso, around the town of Yamaga, is another cluster of popular hot-spring resorts. These springs were discovered more than eight hundred years ago by hunters who observed deer bathing in them. The principal hot springs in the area, most of which are found along the Kikuchi River, are Kikuchi, Yamaga, Awasegawa, Kumairi, Miyabaru, and Hirajima.

HINAGU

Located on the western coast of Kumamoto Prefecture, on the Yashiro Sea, Hinagu is a large and popular resort frequented chiefly by visitors to the scenic Amakusa Islands across Yashiro Bay.

MIYAZAKI PREFECTURE

EBINO PLATEAU DISTRICT

Miyazaki Prefecture, unlike Kumamoto and Oita immediately to the north, has relatively few volcanic springs. The major concentration of hot springs is in the far south, on the Ebino Plateau and along the northern slopes of Mt. Kirishima. Chief *onsen* in the district are Ebino-kogen, Abagahira, Yunomoto, Hasutaro, Shiratori, Kyomachi, and Yoshida.

KAGOSHIMA PREFECTURE

MT. KIRISHIMA DISTRICT

The southern slopes of Mt. Kirishima spill into Kagoshima Prefecture, and are amply supplied with hot springs. The height of the plateaus and foothills of Mt. Kirishima range from about 1,970 feet to 4,590 feet. Principal spas in the region include Shinyu, Hayashida, Iodani, Maruo, Yunotani, and Sekibira.

SHINKAWA DISTRICT

Slightly southwest of Mt. Kirishima is the Shinkawa district of volcanic springs, which is one of the major resort areas of nearby Kagoshima City. The major hot-spring towns are Shiobitashi, Ramune, Yamanoyu, Shinkawa, Anraku, Myoken, and Hinatayama.

IBUSUKI

To the south of Kagoshima City, at the very bottom of the Satsuma Peninsula, is the town of Ibusuki, famed as a honeymoon spot and a popular tourist resort. Like Beppu, Ibusuki boasts a wide variety of geothermal springs, and visitors are drawn as much to the sand baths on the beaches as to the huge indoor "jungle baths." Nearby are the small seaside spas of Narikawa and Kawajiri, which offer beautiful views of the conical Mt. Kaimon across the bay.

*T*he photographs for *Furo* were shot over a period of nearly ten years. A few appeared in two previous books, *Water: A View from Japan* and *Sensual Water*, both of which were created by Bernard Barber and myself. Bernard first suggested that we do a book on the Japanese bath. I am grateful to him for much of the inspiration and many of the ideas in this book and sad that he was not able to work with me on it though his presence is felt and seen.

The pressures and deadlines of working on this book were greatly overshadowed by the pleasures and rewards of working with my longtime friend Peter Grilli. His knowledge of Japan, the Japanese people, and the Japanese language coupled with his enthusiasm and curiosity made the project exciting, educational, and fun.

People often asked how I was able to shoot photographs in the baths. There were two main problems: one climatic, the other social. The first, in a word, was steam. Baths are small, enclosed spaces filled with moisture. It is a tribute to the makers of my cameras (three 35 mm Nikons and a 6x7 Pentax) that they withstood the abuse of hundreds of hot and steamy sessions in bathhouses. Japanese bathers always carry a small towel into the bath which serves three purposes: to cover one's private parts, to wash with, and to dry with. I found a fourth use: to wipe my (filter-covered) lenses and eyepieces, an action that had to be accomplished quickly and repeatedly. I also found it helpful to preheat the camera by letting it sit in a warm room to reach a temperature a little closer to that of the bathroom.

The social problem was—how do you enter someone's very private world, especially as a foreigner with a camera, and not be or appear to be a voyeur? In most cases the solution was quite simple. I always entered the bathroom as did the others, naked and with towel. I followed proper bathroom etiquette, and I talked with my fellow bathers. Then, after some rapport was established, I went to get my camera. As you look through this book you can see that mine was not the only camera in the baths. It was often impossible for me to shoot in the women's baths so I was forced to use telephoto lenses on occasion or to send female friends into the baths in my stead.

One of those friends deserves a very special thank-you. My companion of the bath—and work and life—Tish O'Connor often lured female bathers into the "mixed" baths (usually occupied only by men) and precipitated some wonderful bath parties. By her enthusiasm and persistence she discovered new locations; with her smile and charm, she put shy subjects at ease. As I worked on the design and layout of this book, she was my best critic and suggested numerous solutions which added greatly to its organization and visual impact. On this last page I have the last word and it is for Tish: Thank you, my love.

PETER GRILLI

possesses a rare knowledge of Japan, where he spent his childhood. He took his BA and MA degrees in Japanese history and literature at Harvard University. He was for many years Director of Education, Film and Performing Arts at the Japan Society in New York, and Director of the Japan Project for U.S. public television. He travels frequently to and within Japan, has produced award-winning films and television programs on that country, and currently is active as a consultant and writer specializing on Japanese-American cultural relations.

DANA LEVY

is a book designer and photographer who lived and worked in Japan for seven years. Since his first celebrated work *Bamboo,* he has designed and photographed many books and museum catalogues, including: *Kanban: The Art of the Japanese Shop Sign;* and *Anatomy Illustrated* (winner of the 1980 American Book Award). With his wife Letitia Burns O'Connor, he founded Perpetua Press in Los Angeles, a firm that produces illustrated books for trade and museum publishers, including the National Gallery of Art, the Asia Society, and the University of Washington Press.

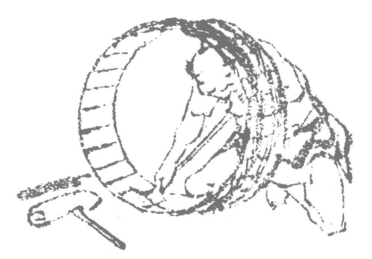

PLEASURES OF THE JAPANESE BATH

Designed by
DANA LEVY

Typeset in Baskerville by
CONTINENTAL TYPOGRAPHICS

Printed in HongKong by
C&C OFFSET PRINTING CO., LTD.